THE BIRTH OF
INDUSTRIAL NURSING

TO

MY MOTHER AND FATHER

WITHOUT WHOSE EARLY TEACHING

WISE EXAMPLE AND UNFAILING ENCOURAGEMENT

THIS BOOK WOULD NEVER HAVE

BEEN WRITTEN

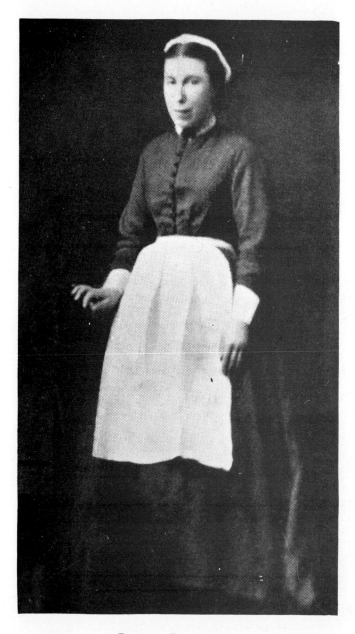

PHILIPPA FLOWERDAY

This frontispiece is reproduced from an old group picture: see page 49

THE BIRTH OF
INDUSTRIAL NURSING

Its History and Development
in Great Britain

BY

IRENE H. CHARLEY
S.R.N., S.C.M., H.V. Cert.

Nursing Consultant, Crusader Insurance Company Limited

WITH A FOREWORD BY

A. A. WOODMAN
M.B.E., S.R.N., S.C.M., H.V. Cert.

Chairman of Council, Royal College of Nursing

BAILLIÈRE TINDALL · LONDON

A BAILLIÈRE TINDALL book published by
Cassell Ltd.
35 Red Lion Square, London WC1R 4SG
and at Sydney, Auckland, Toronto, Johannesburg

an affiliate of
Macmillan Publishing Co. Inc.
New York

© 1978 Baillière Tindall
a division of Cassell Ltd.

First published July 1954

Reprinted and re-issued 1978

ISBN 0 7020 0720 X

Printed in Great Britain by Billing & Sons Limited,
Guildford, London and Worcester.

FOREWORD

THIS book, so obviously written from the heart of the author and telling the history of a social movement, represents on her part no plunge into unknown depths for it is the result of personal experiences and the constant gathering up of material over a number of years. Primarily intended to be of use to those concerned in Occupational Health Services it will remedy somewhat the scarcity of information which has hitherto been available on the historical development of the industrial health movement. It also offers some interesting reading for those who know little of the subject. The accounts that are given of some of the early struggles and of the many outstanding personalities who have contributed towards the astonishing revolution that has occurred will stir the imagination of the reader.

The quotation in the Preface, so aptly taken from the Apocrypha, gives an indication of the author's approach to the subject, for in the book the reader is constantly reminded that during the earlier years spiritual as well as temporal aid for the workers was encouraged by the enlightened and far-seeing employers of the day.

The story of the progression throughout three centuries towards the humanising of industry and the promotion of the health of the workers is a fascinating one and Miss Charley's account of the effects of the recent war, with the large increase in the number of women workers and the rapid development of the health and welfare work within industry which resulted from it, is absorbingly interesting.

Many references are made in the book to the efforts of the Royal College of Nursing to provide post-certificate educational facilities for State registered nurses entering or already engaged in industrial nursing and to the steady pressure exercised by this body towards establishing recognition of this new branch of the profession.

A considerable expansion of the services of the industrial nurse in the near future can be forecast, with the first emphasis on the prevention of illness and the establishment of complete co-ordination of all the social services concerned with the health and general welfare of the community.

A. A. WOODMAN, M.B.E., S.R.N., S.C.M., H.V.Cert.

Chairman of Council,
Royal College of Nursing.

PREFACE

THIS brief history of industrial nursing in Great Britain has been written primarily for nurse students entering industry and those already engaged in the Industrial Nursing Service, but it may also be of interest to others who are concerned in this new branch of the Public Health Nursing Service. It traces some early pioneer influences in the development of industrial health in this country and discusses the social conditions of the population at the time when the industrial nurse was emerging as a specialised public health worker. It describes the awakening of the nurse to the need for professional organisation during the period between the wars and the part that she later played in preparing herself for the wider field of social medicine lying before her.

Although the period under review comes to an end in 1948, a natural break arising from the introduction of the National Health Service, reference is made in the book to the setting up by the Prime Minister of the Dale Committee in 1949. Its findings, which indicate in some ways what progress may be expected in the future, are discussed.

It is realised that this historical survey is by no means exhaustive and that other pioneering nursing influences may have been at work during the last 100 years, evidence of which has not been discovered in the search already made. Little, indeed, is at present known of the early history of industrial nursing. It is hoped, therefore, that the publication of this book will stimulate interest in the subject and that facts not yet generally known, which might add to the comprehensiveness of the review, will be brought to light, so that they may, perhaps, be incorporated in a future edition.

John Masefield, the Poet Laureate, has written: "If there be the will to have a splendid thing that thing will be made. A nation is great in so far as she wills to have splendid things. If she wills them they will come. If she does not she will mess along with anything which will somehow do." Industrial Britain has willed to have " a splendid thing " in the form of an occupational health service for its people and the industrial nurse is playing her part in its development. Industrial nursing may be described as the application of the science and art of nursing to the needs of the worker at his place of employment; it includes activities initiated within industry or commerce on behalf of the worker's health, safety and general well-being; it may be available to the employees only within the factory or office, or it may be extended outside to the employees and their families; it may also co-operate in providing other community activities in the neighbourhood. It is a specialised branch of public health nursing comprising both the principles of sociology and the prevention of occupational disease and accidents, and takes its appropriate place in the wide field of social medicine studying Man in relation to his environment.

The development of this specialised branch of public health nursing in Great Britain is the subject of this book. Many social influences have combined through the years to shape the organisation which now makes it possible for the nurse to make her own contribution to the industrial and commercial world to-day. So wide is her present sphere of influence that she finds herself working in mining and in transport, at sea, in the air and on the quayside, in department stores and hotels, in workshops, in factories and in industry generally.

The historian of public health or social development must try to discover early beginnings and trace them through the ages, and with this object in view it will perhaps be appropriate to quote from the Apocrypha, which was written in the first half of the second century B.C., a delightful description of the industrial worker:

" The wisdom of a learned man cometh by opportunity of leisure; and he that hath little business shall become wise.
" How can he get wisdom that holdeth the plough, and that

glorieth in the goad, that driveth oxen, and is occupied in their labours, and whose talk is of bullocks?

" He giveth his mind to make furrows; and is diligent to give the kine fodder.

" So every carpenter and workmaster, that laboureth night and day; and they that cut and grave seals, and are diligent to make great variety, and give themselves to counterfeit imagery, and watch to finish a work.

" The smith also sitting by the anvil, and considering the iron work, the vapours of the fire wasteth his flesh, and he fighteth with the heat of the furnace; the noise of the hammer and the anvil is ever in his ears, and his eyes look still upon the pattern of the thing that he maketh; he setteth his mind to finish his work, and watcheth to polish it perfectly.

" So doth the potter sitting at his work, and turning the wheel about with his feet, who is always carefully set at his work, and maketh all his work by number;

" He fashioneth the clay with his arm, and boweth down his strength before his feet; he applieth himself to lead it over; and he is diligent to make clean the furnace.

" All these trusts to their hands; and every one is wise in his work.

" Without these cannot a city be inhabited; and they shall not dwell where they will, nor go up and down;

" They shall not be sought for in public counsel, nor sit high in the congregation, they shall not sit on the judges' seat, nor understand the sentence of judgment; they cannot declare justice and judgment; and they shall not be found where parables are spoken.

" But they will maintain the state of the world and (all) their desire is in the work of their craft."

Ecclesiasticus XXXVIII. 24-34.

London,   IRENE H. CHARLEY.
April, 1954.

ACKNOWLEDGMENTS

It is with a deep sense of gratitude that the writer acknowledges the practical help with the writing of this book she has received from a wide circle of colleagues, friends and official sources. To the Factory Department of the Ministry of Labour and National Service and the Controller of H.M. Stationery Office she acknowledges permission to quote extracts from official reports and circulars. She is grateful to the Royal College of Nursing for giving her access to material describing the part the Royal College has played in industrial nursing organisation, and to the executors of the late Sir Arthur Stanley for permission to reproduce letters appearing in *The Times*.

She is indebted to Dr. E. H. Capel, formerly Chief Medical Officer, National Coal Board; Dr. W. E. Chiesman and Dr. C. Roberts of the Treasury Medical Service; Dr. Cavendish Fuller, Chief Medical Officer, British Railways; Air Marshal Sir Harold Whittingham, British Overseas Airways Corporation; Dr. L. G. Norman, Chief Medical Officer, London Transport Executive; and Dr. P. Pringle, Chief Medical Officer, British Electricity Authority, for information concerning the development of industrial nursing in the nationalised industries described in Chapter 10; to the late Miss Ethel Colman for her research about the first industrial nurse, outlined in Chapter 3; to Professor Arthur Raistrick for historical details in Chapter 1; to Mr. C. H. Ward-Jackson for information about the early beginnings of welfare work in Courtaulds Ltd.; to Mrs. C. U. Cole for much material about early welfare work; to Mrs. Mary Agnes Hamilton for permission to quote from her book *Mary Macarthur - a Biographical Sketch*; to the Royal National Mission to Deep Sea Fishermen, the Aberdeen Steam Fisheries Provident Society and the Industrial Christian Fellowship, for permission to describe their early activities; and to the Tees-side Hospital Management

Committee for details of the early days of North Ormesby Hospital, Middlesbrough.

Further acknowledgments are due to the Overseas Food Corporation; to the Institute of Insurance, for material quoted from a report published by them, which appears in Chapter 10; to Miss Clare Sykes, formerly of the Ministry of Supply, for permission to reproduce extracts from her paper given at the Ninth International Industrial Health Congress of the Commission Internationale Permanente pour la Médecine du Travail which was held in London in September, 1948; to Lever Brothers and Unilever Ltd., Whitbreads, Ltd., English Electric Co., Ltd, and the Cray Valley Industrial Association, Ltd., for details about their activities; and to Miss Elizabeth Hopkins, S.R.N., for much help in reading the manuscript and for many practical suggestions.

The author would also like to express her grateful thanks to the Directors of the Crusader Insurance Company Limited for much help and encouragement and for the opportunities given to her to study the industrial nursing service which has been described, and also to Miss J. E. Slocombe for secretarial help. Finally, she wishes to pay tribute to the large number of industrial nurses and factory managements who have created an industrial nursing service over the years and whose story of pioneering effort it has been her pleasure to unfold.

CONTENTS

I

Early Beginnings

TRACES of one of the earliest industries in this country which can be linked with the Roman occupation are still to be found in the Forest of Dean, where scowles holes are to be seen showing the early workings of iron ore and coal.

The Forester, a direct descendant of a sturdy race of independent Britons, is proud of his inheritance and clings tenaciously to the title of Freeminer and all that word implies. The Coal Commission under the Coal Act, 1938, operates in all the coalfields of Great Britain with the exception of the Forest of Dean and even the National Coal Board is not the ultimate authority in matters of coal mining there. In this coalfield these matters are subject to the ancient rights and privileges of the Freeminers. By definition in the Act " Freeminers may now be defined as all male persons born and abiding in the Hundred of St. Briavels of the age of 21 years and upwards who shall have worked a year and a day in a coal or iron ore mine within the Hundred of St. Briavels." The Gaveller, who in olden times was the King's representative, could grant a " gale " or piece of land to a group of four Freeminers, who worked that land and the ore beneath as partners. The King was the fifth partner in each " gale " and the Gaveller had to call at the mine every Tuesday, between Matins and Mass, for the King's share of the profits. The Freeminers today are still granted " gales " and have the right to sell, transfer, assign or dispose of them to others.

Evidently the spiritual needs of these early miners was the

concern of the Church, for a famous fifteenth-century brass to be found in the Greyndour Chantry in All Saints' Church, Newland, portrays a Freeminer dressed for work. This beautiful church is called the Cathedral of the Forest and was founded about 1200. History records that a Chantry anciently called " Our Lady's Service " was founded " to support a priest, called the Morrowe Masse Priest, celebrating at the altar of the Virgin Mary, bound to go from one smithy or mining pit to another within the parish twice a week to say them Gospels." The Morrowe Masse was for those who had to go to work very early. It was sometimes at 5 a.m. The brass in the floor of the Greyndour Chapel shows a Freeminer dressed in a tunic half-way down to his knees, with a hood as head covering. A short-handled pick is in his hand. He has a shaggy beard and a sack slung over his left shoulder. Leather thongs are round the trouser leg. This style of dress was followed in every detail until down to the end of the nineteenth century.

A quaint though somewhat primitive expression of legal opinion in early days is suggested by the law of Deodand which was passed in 1540 and may be quoted as a forerunner of the present Industrial Injuries Act. Cowall says " Deodand is a thing given or rather forfeited, as it were, to God for the pacification of His wrath, in case of misadventure, whereby any Christian man cometh to a violent end, without the fault of any reasonable creature." The law said " Whatever personal chattel is the immediate occasion of the death of any reasonable creature is forfeited to the King to be applied to pious uses and distributed in alms by his high almoner." There is on record the case of a child who, playing near a " horse myll " was killed. Under the law of Deodand the mill was destroyed to " punish " it for having killed the child. Although this was an early legal conception, the act was not abolished until 1845 when the introduction of machinery in industry and the rise of capitalism changed the outlook towards the responsibility of the employer to his workmen. The incident referred to appears in the commonplace book of John Hooker of Exeter in the following quaint phraseology: " A yonge child standing near to the whele of a horse myll was by some mishap come within the swepe of the compasse of the cogge whele. And upon inquisition taken it was founde that the whele was the cause of the childe's deathe, whereupon, the myll was forthwith defaced and pulled down."

Crowley Iron Undertakings.

One of the earliest references to industrial health services in Great Britain comes from Sussex, where the Crowley Iron Undertakings, in the sixteenth century, administered a joint health plan which was supported voluntarily by masters and men. The work of this firm was done partly in its own forges and partly by small groups whom the Crowleys supplied with iron for making ships' anchors. A clergyman and schoolmaster were employed and a doctor was available in case of accidents, but little more is known of this pioneer activity.

London (Quaker) Lead Company.

To Professor Arthur Raistrick, M.Sc., Ph.D., F.G.S., M.I.Min.E., King's College, Newcastle upon Tyne, Professor of Mining, Durham University, we are indebted for many interesting facts about one of the earliest and most comprehensive health services of which records are available. In his book *Two Centuries of Industrial Welfare, The London (Quaker) Lead Company, 1692-1905*, with sub-titles *The Social policy and work of the Governors and Company for smelting down lead with pit coal and sea coal mainly in Alston Moor and the Pennines*, are recorded many of the activities which developed in a small lead mining community in the Pennines, and a point worthy of note is that the miners themselves first formed an organisation known as " The Society of Miners " and developed a complete medical and social club the benefits extending to their families. The Society was later taken over by the firm. There is a mention in the ancient records that the Company sent a woman to train as a midwife, later to return to work in the mining villages.

Interesting extracts from this book read:

From its information, the Company had been careful for the miners' general health. During the nineteenth century much thought and money was spent on promoting miners' welfare and medical benefit societies, with the co-operation of the men. During the eighteenth century the miners of Alston Moor banded themselves together in an association approximating to a Friendly Society, and this later was absorbed into the Company's welfare fund and schemes. The Society was based on regular subscriptions, with graded benefits for ill health, accident, and death, and had a very comprehensive set of rules and orders, many of which are of special interest and some of rather humorous aspect.

This Society of Miners of Alston Moor was one of the earliest of the Friendly Societies that sprang up during the Industrial Revolution, but was by no means unique.

The Company laid down very strict rules for the guidance of the conduct of their doctors, and for the conduct of the funds, and in 1829 decided to codify all their various rules, and supply them in the contract of appointment. The rules are as follows:

Rules and Regulations

to be observed by the medical gentlemen in the employment of

The Lead Company

To Mr....................

Sir,

You having been appointed Medical Attendant to the Workmen in the employment of the Governor and Company, I am directed by the Court of Directors to call your attention to the following instructions:

I am, Sir,

your obedient servant,

Middleton House 18 ....

You are to attend upon all the afflicted members and their families residing within your district, as often as the nature of the complaint may require, and supply them with and send them such medicine, etc, as the nature of their afflictions require; and in case of accident or sudden dangerous illness, you must visit, or procure a person, properly qualified, to visit such member, by night or by day, *with all convenient speed*, and render all the assistance you, or such medical practitioner is capable of rendering. And you shall hold your office so long as you discharge the duties, and perform the engagements to the Company with fidelity, honour, and to the satisfaction of the Court.

For those men who are Members of the Workmen's Fund, you must sign the Certificate which the affiliated member is to send, each month, for his money, every time you visit him; and it is essentially necessary, for the information and guidance of the Committee, that you do always, at your first visit, write the nature of the member's complaint on his sickness paper; and on the back thereof, the state of the member's health upon each subsequent visit, the date of which is to be inserted.

You are to visit personally, at their own homes, the sick members, immediately you are required to do so, as it will occur that the progress of fever may be arrested, and its otherwise regular course prevented by timely assistance.

And in internal inflammation, so prevalent among the working classes, the important period of a few hours being lost for blistering or bleeding, fatal consequences ensue, rendering all future attempts at remedying fruitless.

In case of accident, also, the prompt assistance of a medical gentleman will, of course, frequently prevent after mischiefs and tedious complaints.

You are never to require members of the sick fund to attend at your residence, for advice, nor the sickness paper to be brought there for signature, and to be particular that all medicines, etc. furnished to them, are carefully labelled.

(Those persons only who do not declare on the fund for the sick relief, or, if not members of the fund, whose diseases are trivial, to be required to wait on the medical gentlemen for medicine or advice.)

You must impress on the sick members the proper regimen

to be observed for their complaints; and when it may be conducive to their health, you must prescribe, distinctly, the hours of the day during which it will be really beneficial for them to take the air.

And in your visits and intercourse with the members and their families, you must bear in mind that not only prompt personal attendance, *but the highest degree of courtesy and kindness of manner* is requisite towards them, they being, generally, more susceptible to slights than persons of more liberal education, and of the higher walks of life.

Lastly, the Court wish to impress upon you the consequences which must arise, if members (who are not apt to declare on the sick fund too early, but rather otherwise), be slightingly attended to or a trifling medicine sent them by an assistant, or from neglect to label medicines with the proper directions, and not impressing on sick members the best regimen to be observed, etc.—diseases will be protracted, or disorders confirmed, to the danger of life—to the serious injury of the workmen's fund—and protracted attendance of the medical gentlemen themselves.

London, 26th March, 1829.

. . . .

The accident record of the Company, in comparison with general figures for the industry at that time, was low and this was largely due to the fact that in each district mine captains were appointed by the Company who were responsible for the safety in all working places. An accident record appearing in the Company's books in 1852 might be duplicated in official mines reports today: " 1852. John Allison, killed, Ashgill Head Mine, level, contrary to regulation, riding in the waggon."

When the Nent Head estate was developed and the new village created, a school was held in the Company's office, with a proper schoolmaster to take care of the miners' children, the schoolmaster probably being paid by the children's school pence. At the same time the Company established Sunday Schools, again to be held in their office buildings. It was a condition of employment by the Company that a miner's children should attend the school regularly, as well as attending Sunday School and a place of worship each week. Boys were to attend the schools from the age of six years to twelve years, and girls from six years to fourteen years. The schools reflect the spirit of the times in their continual insistence on religious and moral training as their prime duty. Libraries had been provided from the earliest days of the Company in the Friends' Meeting Houses built in all the mining areas, but the books provided there were entirely confined to religious works, journals of Friends, etc.

Bernardino Ramazzini, the Father of Industrial Medicine.
Although it cannot be claimed that the work of Ramazzini had a direct influence on industrial health in this country, yet it is mentioned here because in his writings the inclusion of midwifery as a dangerous calling will be of interest to industrial nurses who are also midwives but may not have realised that their own work was once fraught with a danger equal to that experienced by some of their industrial patients today. Furthermore, he compares the hazards of the midwife working in Italy with those in England, France, and Germany. Ramazzini —an Italian Professor of Medicine at Modena, living from 1633 to 1714—published in Latin *Diseases of Tradesmen and Craftmen* and in relation to midwives he says in Chapter XIX:

> " Though midwives do not incur such danger by assisting women in childbirth as the bearers do in interring a corpse, yet they do not always escape free when they receive the birth together with the flux which comes from the uterus. I need not mention the corruption of the lochia, the diminution or suppression of the whole flux for a few hours is enough to kill the woman who lies in. Pliny says: ' The mentrual flux has such noxious qualities that it sours alum, blasts corn, kills what comes anear it and burns the fruits of the earth! ' "
> " Now the midwives standing ready to receive the birth with

expanded hands and continuing in that posture for several hours, receive no small damage to their very hands from the dropping of the lochia, insomuch that sometimes their hands are ulcerated by the sharp corrosive matter. So that as a nurse who suckles a foul child receives the first infection in the breasts."

" This your expert and prudent midwives are fully aware of, for when they are obliged to lay a pocky woman they wrap their hands up in linen cloths and wash them often in water and vinegar."

" Add to all this that the midwives receive at the mouth and nostrils the noxious steam arising from the flux of the womb, and which is yet worse, they cannot arm themselves against them with sweet scented odours, these being apt to throw the woman in labour into hysteric fits."

" Perhaps the women midwives are not so much exposed to danger in England, France and Germany where the women bring forth their children in bed and not upon perforated stools as they do in Italy. In fine the midwives that would perform their office without the dangers of infection ought every now and then when they have respite, to wash their hands in water and vinegar and shift themselves. And in a word they ought to take nice care all along to have clean things about them. A certain old midwife told me that when she was called to tend a pocky or cachectic woman she used to stay to the very last throes before she set her upon the stool by which means she kept her hands from being so long exposed to the dropping of the contagious lochia."

Diseases of Tradesmen and Craftsmen is described as a dissertation on endemial diseases or those disorders which arise from particular climates, situations and methods of living, together with a " Treatise on the Diseases of Tradesmen to which they are subject by their particular callings with the method of avoiding and treating them."

It is worthy of note that Ramazzini suggested no profit should be made out of labour leading to highly dangerous diseases, his words being: " The worst profit is that which is gained in destroying health, the most precious of all goods." This exhaustive work, which remains an outstanding classic, describes the diseases of a wide variety of industries ranging from stone cutters, millers, masons, bricklayers, pickers of hemp, flax, silk, salt pits, learned men, grooms, chemists, potters, glassmakers, painters, brimstone, blacksmiths, workers in lime and plaster of paris, apothecaries, fullers, fanners, metal diggers, gilders, surgeons, to wet nurses.

James Lind in the Royal Navy.

In 1756 James Lind, a doctor in the Royal Navy, published *A Treatise Upon the Scurvy*. It is an enquiry into the nature, causes and cure of that disease and is a landmark in the history of preventive medicine. The diet and general living conditions of the sailors in those days were indescribably terrible. Potatoes and salt pork made their staple diet although Dr. Lind records that he always provided sundry casks of apples, believing firmly that they prevented scurvy. Morbidity and mortality from the disease in the Navy were alarmingly high. Certain elderly and infirm seamen were employed as sick bay attendants and were trained chiefly to use a tourniquet to stop haemorrhage, this first-aid measure being in constant demand owing to the primitive surgery practised in those days. Lind observed that after being in port at Gibraltar, or other stations where fresh fruit and vegetables were taken on board, scurvy disappeared on his ship only to reappear again after some time at sea when the stocks were exhausted.

About the same period another young surgeon in the Fleet, John Knyveton, whose interesting diary was published under the title *Surgeon's Mate*, observed similiar conditions among his sailors, and the introduction of citrus fruit to their diet controlled the situation and laid the foundation for modern dietary reforms in the Navy.

John Smedley.

From Smedley's *Practical Hydropathy*, first published in 1857, a quaint and fascinating volume throwing considerable light on the health activities in a cotton mill in Derbyshire, can be gleaned something of the concern one employer in this district showed for his workpeople. John Smedley, the owner of Lea Mills, one mile from Cromford Station, Derbyshire, the author of the book, tells, in the characteristic literary style of that age, of his pioneering efforts to develop hydropathy in this country. Conscience no doubt was responsible for the fact that in retirement he could find no repose of mind—he saw himself as a hypocrite, but later, through the help of some of his workpeople he found " peace in believing ". He laboured in visiting the poor and the schools and practised self-denial of those extravagances he formerly rejoiced in.

At Lea Bridge, his home, he took in a few men upon whom to try hydropathic remedies; later places for free board, lodging and baths for males and females were arranged. He bought a small house at Matlock Bank for six patients, where board, lodging and treatment at 3s. a day was given. This developed into the Hydropathic Establishment at Matlock Bath. Mrs. Smedley was responsible for the domestic arrangements of the establishment and *Mrs. Smedley's Manual* giving recipes for beef steaks and cutlets, new milk jellies for invalids and pomade for the hair, may still be referred to as a guide to invalid cookery. One of the principal objects Smedley had in view in this work was to teach hydropathic remedies for self-application and to show the labouring classes how to carry out many of the processes with the simple means within their reach. Supplies of baths, bandages, and any appliances named in the book could be had on application to the Manager at Lea Mills. Furthermore, mustard bran for foot baths could be had, free of charge, at Lea Mills by the working people.

It must not be imagined that the introduction of these new methods was not challenged by " orthodox medicine " of that day and a study of this book is of considerable interest in this respect as this doughty pioneer seeks to justify his somewhat empirical methods. Today his practices might be frowned upon, as the following description of a factory accident suggests: " Case of a man burnt with molten lead—the lead went into both eyes, over face, one hand and wrist and caused excruciating pain. Smedley's special hydropathic treatment was immediately given by means of some boiling water in a vessel with a narrow board put across it for the affected hand to rest upon and so have the benefit of the steam. Then a thick woollen wrapper thrown over the man's hand and vessel altogether so to keep in the steam, every five minutes just lifting the wrapper up and gently putting into the vessel a few red hot cokes out of the fire nicely kept up the steam. This process soon eased the pain by setting eyes, nose and mouth watering well, which drew away the inflammation gradually as well as the pain. Steaming and poultices were repeated at night. Next day the patient was partially able to work and the following day was quite restored, the eyes only being sponged with milk and water."

Smedley suggested employers should make it possible to use a very simple plan of bathing, by appropriating a room for the purpose, with a few sitz baths, one or two shallow baths, a steamer, some sponges, and sheets. He offered to furnish articles at cost price and sent an experienced man to give instructions in their use. He maintained the treatment would soon repay the expense incurred, by making the workman more capable of performing his duties with efficiency. He believed so much in this policy, both as a duty and from an economic point of view, that he provided his workpeople with a complete hydropathic department, and a cooking-house and servants for preparing meals. Scotch oatmeal porridge with golden syrup or milk for fivepence per week was in the menu. He gave his factory "hands" an additional half-hour each morning for religious worship and for hearing any important events going on in the world. All the 350 employees assembled in a room in the winter, and in a marquee during the summer, from half past eight to nine. His philosophy taught that by these means the mind and body is refreshed. He thought, if given time for reflection, men are made for nobler purposes than merely working for the support of the body. He prophesied there was a time approaching in which there would be no avaricious or unfeeling " masters ", not any thoughtless or indifferent to the welfare of those around them, and when the factory " hand " would be found amongst the highest.

North Ormesby Hospital.

In *A Brief Story of the Development of North Ormesby Hospital* an interesting tale is told how in 1858 John Jordison, a Middlesbrough postmaster and printer, convinced Sister Mary Rachel Jaques of the Sisterhood of the Holy Rood that the growing town of Middlesbrough, with a population of 15,000 souls, offered a suitable sphere for her labours, and how this need was made tragically realistic by a serious accident which occurred at the Ironworks of Snowdon Hopkins & Co. One of the stationary boilers that supplied steam for the working of the rolling mills and steam hammer burst with a tremendous report. Sixteen or seventeen men were injured by flying debris and by escaping steam, and several were blown into the river. There was no hospital or infirmary nearer than Newcastle. Some of the injured were sent there and two of them died on the way. Some were taken to their own homes or lodgings and two were laid in a stable belonging to the Ship Inn in Stockton Street. This stable, built on an open stall, rose and fell with the tide, which carried with it all the impurities of that end of Middlesbrough. It being the middle of summer, the smell was almost unbearable. One man was taken to Dacre Street, where the bed took fire and had to be dragged from under him. He was then laid upon a heap of straw despite his open wounds. Another man was so burnt and scalded by steam that the oil and limewater dressing was absorbed.

It was into this maelstrom and squalor of industrial development that Sister Mary came, having but recently returned from the Deaconesses Institution in Kaiserswerth where Florence Nightingale had previously been prepared for her great and noble work. In the beginning Sister Mary attended to the needs of the sufferings in their own homes or lodgings. It should be remembered that at this time in the history of Middlesbrough the population ratio was ten males to one female and that life had few refinements or gentle influences. The story goes on to tell of the purchase of a house in Albert Road, Middlesbrough, and of two cottages immediately behind in Dundas Mews. Passages were constructed linking the house to the cottages. Sister Mary and two nurses lived in the house and the original Cottage Hospital was established and opened in the spring of the year 1859.

It should be remembered that employees' contributions—the system of weekly contributions by working men for the maintenance of local hospitals—were initiated at Middlesbrough, and by these means the foundation of the Cottage Hospital was well and truly set; Sister Mary Jaques and the Sisters of the Holy Rood provided the nursing care in the " wards ". Though first steps had been taken, these were soon to prove unequal to meet the needs of the growing population of Middlesbrough. Two more cottages were taken, but soon four cottages were inadequate. Sister Mary later relinquished her work in Middlesbrough to establish a home for incurables in London. Sister Elizabeth carried on the work of the hospital, later to be known as the North Ormesby Hospital, as Sister-in-Charge and acted as Mother Superior from 1870-1905. Many are the stories told of her. She was known as " The Angel in the House " and the story is related of an old Irishman who, having said good-bye to her at the top of the stairs, went down a few steps, stopped and looked round, and supposing no eye saw his movement, mounted the steps again, knelt down and kissed the spot where she had stood. The handsome stained glass window provided to her memory by public subscription still adorns the beautiful entrance hall of the hospital.

The name of another nursing pioneer must be mentioned in relation to industrial development in the Midlands. Sister

Dora of Walsall was the youngest daughter of the Reverend Mark James Pattison, Rector of Haukswell, Yorkshire. In those early days it was a courageous act at the age of thirty-two to join, against the wishes of her family, the Sisterhood of the Good Samaritans at Coathan in Yorkshire. Later Sister Dora came to Walsall to work in the small Cottage Hospital there. In October 1875 there was a devastating explosion at Birchell's Ironworks. Men were horribly burned with the molten metal and dressing their wounds was a procedure from which the doctors and nurses shrank. But Sister Dora, ever calm and capable, gave skilful service to the tortured bodies and nursed them night and day. Sister Dora died in 1878 and the first statue to a woman ever erected in Britain was unveiled to her memory on the bridge at Walsall in 1886.

*A Service on the High Seas.**

It was in 1881 that attention was drawn to the desperate conditions of fishermen in the fleet known as the "Short Blue" owned by Messrs. Hewitt and Company, trawling in the North Sea round the Dogger Bank, a fishing centre extending 120 miles north and south and 65 miles east and west.

A description of the fisherman's life brings to mind the peculiar problems in this, one of the most important industries in the country. At the age of sixteen he signs on as a fisherman and from then onwards his entire life, with the exception of an occasional 36-hour port call or an unwelcome spell of unemployment, will be spent at sea. There are no comforts aboard a steam trawler. When the fisherman gets a few hours of sleep in a hard bunk hardly bigger than himself this is the greatest comfort he knows. The rest of the time is filled with hard and hazardous toil. When fish is plentiful or the weather rough he cannot be spared time for sleep. He must work on while there is work to be done. A gale blows up. It is impos-

---

* These notes were kindly supplied by the Royal National Mission to Deep Sea Fishermen.

sible to run for shelter when the nearest land is hundreds of miles away. The eggshell of a ship must be kept to her course. Mountainous waves break over her. Every hand is needed. Drenched, blinded, chilled by rain and icy spray the men carry on, perhaps for days and nights on end, without sleep, virtually clinging to their jobs on a slippery treacherous deck which threatens to shoot them overboard at any moment. Occasionally it succeeds. Another family is bereaved and to the Government statistics another digit is added. Injuries come as a matter of course. Every fisherman can expect three of these a year. If he is lucky they will be merely crushed fingers or toes or salt sores. If he isn't so lucky he may break a limb or get an internal injury. Trawlers are not built for sick men. Unspeakable suffering may have to be borne before first aid or medical assistance can be obtained.

It was to bring some measure of comfort to these brave men that Mr. E. J. Mather began his work which later developed into the Royal National Mission to Deep Sea Fishermen. Determined to see for himself the conditions prevailing he made a voyage with the fishing fleet and soon decided that a special mission was needed to minister to the men. Apart from the primitive conditions of living, the exposure, the continual physical strain, and the coarseness of food (chiefly salt beef and ship's biscuits), the entire absence of sanitation, first aid equipment, or telegraph communication, there was the daily peril involved in transferring the catch to the carrier ship in mid-ocean. Hardly a day would pass without somebody having a finger or an arm crushed between the trawler and the boat as the waves tossed them together. But what was, perhaps, the final factor in deciding Mr. Mather to press toward the founding of a mission for fishermen was his introduction to the activities of the Dutch " copers " or trading ships. These ships would join the British fishing fleet ostensibly to sell duty free tobacco and other necessary oddments. Actually their principal cargo was rum and raw spirits. The fishermen would go aboard, buy tobacco and then be tempted to drink. Men would become mad drunk and going on till their money was all spent would even barter away the ship's gear for more liquor. Now and then a man would get a fit of delirium tremens and throw himself overboard.

In the early days of the Mission volunteers were accepted to work in the mission ships and such eminent medical men as Sir Wilfred Grenfell and Sir Fredrick Treves are remembered with gratitude and admiration. The spiritual needs of the fishermen were of equal concern to the Mission and in 1882 the first Mission ship carrying Bibles, literature, supplies of woollen clothing, tobacco and a fully equipped medicine chest set out on her maiden voyage. At first it was necessary for the Mission ships to buy their tobacco at a foreign port to enable them to sell at a price that would compete with the " copers ". Later, through the co-operation of Messrs. W. D. and H. O. Wills of Bristol, tobacco was supplied at rates which made it possible for the competition to be met. Later still the Board of Trade was approached and so the way was paved to provide tobacco duty free to British fishermen. As the Mission ships increased the " copers " began to disappear, until in 1887 the Hague Convention finally prohibited the sale of spirits on the high seas. The " Sir Edward P. Wills II " is a first-aid boat belonging to the Mission and has a fully equipped dispensary and sick bay with two swinging cots on board. In emergency it stands by, ready to render any necessary aid on the spot. Should serious injury occur the patient is taken aboard and carried to shore with all speed. This boat moves round the coast following the herring fleet.

Aberdeen Steam Fishers' Provident Society.

From Aberdeen comes the story of a Service which commenced as the result of a tragedy to the trawling fleet in nearby waters.

It was in the year 1900 that a severe gale swept the East

Coast of Scotland and as a result many Aberdeen trawlers foundered and their crews perished. A few years previously a similiar disaster had befallen the Aberdeen fleet and a public subscription had been opened to alleviate the distress and want amongst the dependants of those who had lost their lives. By the time the second disaster befell the fleet, however, this fund was practically exhausted and it was felt that something more than dependence on public sympathy was necessary in order to safeguard the interests of the fishermen and their wives and children against recurrent disasters. With this aim in view, a number of public-spirited men connected with the town and the fishing industry conceived a scheme whereby each fisherman, in return for a contribution of one penny for each day at sea, would be insured against loss of life in course of employment.

As is often the case in these affairs, opposition was experienced from different factions, but in the face of all difficulties the confidence of these men in the enterprise was endorsed by the fishermen, and the Aberdeen Steam Fishers' Provident Society was established. Throughout the preliminary negotiations necessary for the commencement of the Society and during the years of its existence the name of Sir John H. Irwin, K.B.E., trawler owner, has been prominent in the conduct of its affairs. Under his guidance the work of the Society flourished and expanded, and from a modest beginning the Society increased in influence until it is now regarded as an integral part of the industry. The Society provides death benefits for widows and children of members, a comprehensive service of treatment and benefit in case of accident, and benefit for permanent disablement. Treatment is provided in a well-equipped surgery and the Society employs a part-time medical officer and an industrial nursing sister. The Society also arranges for private x-ray examination of members when necessary. Rehabilitation in the Society's gymnasium, radiant heat and infra-red treatments are other benefits enjoyed by members, and every effort is made by the staff, supported by the Committee of Management, to provide the most modern methods of treatment.

Debenham Limited.

It was usual in the early days, when the distributive trades were being concentrated in large stores and multiple shops, for all apprentices and " hands " to live in, the employer being responsible for the board and lodging, and both the leisure and working hours of his employees. This method carried with it a duty to provide some standard of " mothering " for the young people and a Matron was appointed in certain cases to fulfil this function.

To the Army and Navy Stores and Debenham Limited can be given the credit for being the first to provide health supervision to their employees. In 1872 a Medical Officer was appointed by the Army and Navy Stores and shortly afterwards a similiar appointment was made by Debenham Limited. Two part-time doctors were appointed by this firm, their attendance at the Medical Department providing routine medical supervision. Later, State-registered Nurses were appointed to assist them. All absentees through sickness or minor ailments reported to the Department and were passed by the doctor before returning to work. In the case of one day's absence through illness the nurse could give permission to return to work.

These arrangements were shared by Debenham and Freebody Ltd., Marshall and Snelgrove Ltd., and Debenham Ltd. All employees in the shops, restaurants, canteens, offices, fire service, despatch and cleaning departments were eligible to make use of the Service. There were about 4,000 employees in all.

At this time the apprentice system was still working both for showrooms and workrooms. All the young people were medically examined before employment. The showroom girls and "matchers" were also tested for colour blindness. The examination required by the Home Office was combined with that given by the doctor employed by the firm. A lady doctor was available for those who preferred to be examined by a woman and a certain number took advantage of this privilege. This service was also shared by Harvey Nicholls Ltd., who sent the young people for examination by arrangement.

Debenham Limited administered their own Approved Society which any members of the firm could join. After leaving employment with the company membership could be continued. The benefits given were usually generous and membership was appreciated although a medical examination was necessary before admission. Vaccination was compulsory and was done by the doctors. Prophylactic injections were also given for the prevention of colds. The nursing staff was responsible for the routine administration of the Medical Department and for all duties in connection with the first treatment of minor ailments or accidents. They visited sick employees in their own homes, arranged for hospital appointments and convalescent care and many other services arising out of their patients' needs. Complete medical records were kept, this being an unusually up-to-date procedure at this time. The nurses were also available for emergencies which might happen to customers in the shops.

The workroom apprentices went to the Barret Street Trade School about three days a week, where English, dressmaking and physical training were included in their curriculum. Other big London firms also sent their young people there for a regular period of continued education though this was not always popular as they felt more or less isolated from the others who were full-time students of the school. However although this system was a continuation of the original arrangement for part-time education of young people in industry, yet it may be considered a forerunner of the part-time education now being provided more generally under the recent Education Acts.

Mardon, Son and Hall, Limited.

Few details are available describing the early beginnings of industrial nursing in general manufacturing firms but it is known that in 1896 a surgery was first opened at No. 1 Factory of Mardon, Son and Hall Ltd., boxmakers, Bristol. Miss Hilda Musselwhite, who was a midwife, was known as " Matron " and is remembered as a cheerful, happy woman with outstanding ability, characteristics needed in any pioneer venture in its experimental stage. A thousand girls were employed in this factory and 500 in a branch nearby.

The surgery was opened only two days a week. From the beginning the factory ambulance brigade, to which dispensers were attached, was well organised and the service was administered by Dr. Frederick St. John Bullen, who was full time Medical Officer. A feature of the social work which was an integral part of the medical service was the facilities offered to the girls to run recreational clubs and in this the nurses were active. A games mistress was later employed, this being considered a most advanced step, though its wisdom cannot be doubted when the type of womanhood entering factory work at that time is considered. Little relaxation was provided for women in those days and their life was hard, but the wide interpretation placed by the firm on the meaning of welfare work contributed to the results which have been achieved over the years. It is characteristic of this service that the nurses have always taken some part in the " off-duty " activities of the girls and these have ranged widely over recreational and cultural pursuits.

Later another factory was opened and Miss Perry, trained at the Bristol General Hospital, was appointed as Matron. Mrs. Barbara Lewis, who was trained at Bristol Royal Infirmary, joined the staff in 1911 and her long industrial nursing career was unbroken until retirement in 1937 when she was succeeded by her daughter Kathleen who, to many of the older employees, is still known as " Mrs. Lewis's daughter ".

On the introduction of the first National Insurance Act in 1911 an interesting link was established between the Factory Medical Service and the Bristol Insurance Committee, the firm acting as agents for the administration of the Act. One full-time and two visiting doctors were then employed by the firm and employees could elect to be placed on the " panel " of these doctors. In this way the routine medical service given by the regular "panel" doctors was available and the facilities of the factory surgery were at the disposal of doctors and patients alike, a convenience much appreciated. The nurses were also able to follow up the sick in their own homes to give nursing care if necessary. This useful co-operation existed until July 1948, when nationalisation of the Health Service came into force. Much can be said for the spirit which inspired this early experiment and the results may yet be studied as a model on which a future occupational health service might be fashioned.

2

The Industrial Revolution

AT the beginning of the eighteenth century, iron founding was still a rural industry scattered over the Sussex Weald, the Forest of Dean and along the mountain streams of Yorkshire, Derbyshire, Shropshire and South Wales where wood and water power were plentiful. The name of Crowley, iron founders in Sussex, appears in any description of early industrialisation in this country and later this firm was responsible for pioneer welfare plans which were sponsored for their miners.

Coalbrookdale in Shropshire had become the site of a famous foundry and Arthur Young in his *Annals of Literature* written in 1776 describes it as follows: " Coalbrookdale is a very romantic spot, it is a winding glen between two immense hills which break into various forms and all thickly covered with wood forming the most beautiful sheets of hanging wood. Indeed too beautiful to be much in unison with that variety of horrors art has spread at the bottom; the noise of the forges, mills etc., with all their vast machinery, the flames bursting from the furnaces with the burning of the coal and the smoke of the lime kilns are altogether sublime and would unite well with craggy and bare rocks like St. Vincents at Bristol."

However, the artistic temperament saw a new beauty in the roaring blast from the furnaces and the massive simplicity of Coalbrookdale, attracted artists of the day who have since become famous and fortunately have left on their canvasses a precious heritage, giving an impression of the early industrialism of the country. In the works of John Sell Cotman, Turner and George Robertson, each of whom, taking the foundry as his subject, painted a masterpiece, we see a vivid stirring of the imagination inspired by the strange changes taking place in the countryside. Perhaps Turner's oil painting of Newcastle-upon-Tyne, painted in 1823, is the outstanding picture of that age giving an impression of industrialisation generally, which by that time had become concentrated on the Tyneside.

During those early years Britain was rapidly changing economically and socially and many of her fair valleys and river banks in the North were disfigured by the growing tide of factory buildings and soaring chimneys. No longer could the Englishman and his family provide all their physical needs by the work of their hands on the land or in the home where the spinning wheel and loom were a necessary part of the cottage furniture. Industry was being centralised in mills on the banks of streams, as waterpower was necessary, and the work-people, losing much of their independence, sought work where scientific and mechanical inventions were changing the population from an entirely agricultural peasantry to an industrial community. In less than a century a complete change was brought about in the economic structure of the countryside and history records how rapid was this social revolution.

The first large factory in England was the silk mill George Sorocold built for John and Thomas Lombe at Derby in 1718-22. It is described as follows in the third edition of Defoe's *Tour of Great Britain*, published in 1742:

" Here is a Curiosity of a very extraordinary Nature, and the only one of the Kind in England; I mean those Mills on the Derwent, which work the three capital Italian Engines for making Organzine or Thrown Silk, which, before these Mills were erected, was purchased by English Merchants with ready money in Italy; by which invention one Hand will twist as much Silk, as before could be done by Fifty, and that in a much truer and better manner. This Engine contains 26,586 Wheels, and 96,746 Movements, which work 73,726 Yards of Silk Thread, every time the Water-wheel goes round, which is three times in one minute, and 318,504,960 Yards in one Day and Night. One Water-wheel gives Motion to all the rest of the Wheels and Movements, of which any one may be stopt separately. One Fire-engine, likewise, conveys warm Air to every individual Part of the Machine, and the whole Work is governed by one Regulator. The House which contains this Engine is of a vast Bulk, and Five or Six Stories high."

After this pioneer experiment other silk mills were built at Derby, Belper, Cromford, Stockport and Macclesfield, but as silk was a luxury trade many were later converted into cotton mills, where cheaper articles of clothing could be manufactured both for the home market and for abroad.

In 1730 spinning was first developed by machinery and Watt's discovery of steam in 1740 led to more rapid production in the mills. Hargreaves's Spinning Jenny and Arkwright's water frame, together with Crompton's Spinning Mule, evolving during the next 20 years, were a natural sequence. At first mill machinery was made of wood, later partly of wood and iron, and not until 1784 was an all iron plant made and installed in the Albion Mill, London, by John Rennie, a famous engineer. The chimneys belching forth their blinding smoke among the hills of Lancashire and the West Riding of Yorkshire were an unhappy augury for child life in England.

Because of these changes child labour was growing more and more valuable. Employers seeking a cheap article and small fingers to work the machines, bargained with the Poor Law Guardians in London, Manchester and other large towns and children were sold to the mill-owners in thousands. A proportion of imbecile children was included with the normal ones and the story of Oliver Twist vividly describes the slavery to which these apprentices were subjected.

There are records that women " gamps " were employed in the factories in these early days, one of their duties being to wake the children, dress them, and see they were on duty at 5 a.m. Although it is not suggested that this type of woman can in any way be described as a pioneer in industrial welfare yet, for historical purposes, it should be mentioned that the employers even then provided a service of sorts, although judged by modern standards it could only be described as cruel and inhuman. Fourteen to eighteen hours a day were worked and little people as young as 5 and 6 were employed.

The first effort to improve the lot of these unfortunate children was an " Act for the preservation of the Health and Morals of Apprentices, and others employed in cotton and other mills and cotton and other factories " of 1802, introduced into the first Sir Robert Peel's parliament. This Act applied to all factories employing three or more apprentices or twenty or more other persons. The walls and ceilings of such factories were to be whitewashed twice a year with quicklime and the windows space had to be sufficient to give adequate ventilation. Visitors to the mills were to be appointed by the Justices of the Peace, who could direct the adoption of such sanitary regulations as they thought fit. One of these was to be a magistrate and the other a clergyman. They were to make a periodical written report to quarter sessions on the conditions of the mills.

If infectious disease occurred the visitors were empowered to call in a doctor, the medical fees to be paid by the mill owner. The conditions under which the apprentices worked must have been very undesirable, because the provisions of the Act laid down the following standards: no apprentice must work more than twelve hours a day; no night work was allowed; a suit of clothing must be supplied annually to each apprentice; separate sleeping accommodation must be provided for boys and girls and not more than two in a bed; a " discreet and proper person " paid by the millowner must be employed as a teacher in reading, writing and arithmetic; a room must be set aside for lessons. The apprentices were to be instructed and examined in the principles of the Christian religion for at least one hour on Sundays. An examination by the Vicar of all children of the Church of England faith was required annually, and between the ages of fourteen and eighteen they were to be prepared for confirmation. A register of factories was established and copies of the Act were to be hung in a place easy of access to the workers. The Act was value-less, however, as there were no Inspectors to enforce it.

Soon the problem of child labour in the textile mills became acute. The " apprentices " system was fading away and the " free " children from the neighbourhood around the factory were manning the mills. " Gentlemen," said Robert Owen, speaking in the House in a debate on this problem, " if parish apprentices were formerly deemed worthy of the care of Parliament, I trust you will not withhold from the unpro-tected children of the present day an equal measure of mercy." Owen had practised in his own mill at New Lanark what he was now preaching in Parliament. He had established schools for children from 3 years of age and upwards; the curri-culum included reading, writing and arithmetic and the children were encouraged to play and dance. No child under ten worked in his mills and the children's hours were reduced to twelve.

In 1818 Peel introduced a Bill to amend the Act of 1802. It was to apply to all cotton, woollen, flax and other mills. In many respects it followed the principles laid down by its predecessor with one important exception. The magistrates were to appoint properly qualified persons who were to receive " a full and adequate compensation for their trouble and expenses " from the county rates. A Select Committee under the Chairmanship of Sir Robert Peel himself sat and examined witnesses, including medical men and manufacturers. The point of view of the workers was not heard. Opinion was sharply divided on the effect of factory labour on children. The doctors were, however, unanimous in confirming that " long hours and close confinement were injurious to health and would cause stunted growth and physical deformity, rickets, mesenteric obstruction, weakness of body and imbecility of mind, feverish disorders and general debility."

The Bill laid down that no child under the age of nine should be employed in the cotton mills and there should be no night work. Lord Stanley protested vehemently, maintaining that the Bill interfered with free] labour. It would destroy the cotton trade, children would be dismissed and there would be suffering both among the children and their parents in consequence. "Be cautious what you are about," he said. "If you interfere now in this instance with the regulation of labour, you will find it difficult to find out when to stop." The Bill was, however, passed and sent to the Lords, where another committee was set up under the chairmanship of Lord Kenyon and the evidence heard again. There was a surprising change in the attitude of the medical men who gave evidence on behalf of the employers in opposition to the Bill. From Manchester a Dr. Holme said he had first noticed an increase in contagious fever in 1796 and he thought this was due to double sets of workers being employed, the infection being spread by relays of children sleeping in the same beds. He observed, however, that night workers were not more unhealthy than day workers. He was not prepared to admit that even 23 hours of work would be inconsistent with health.

A Dr. Whatton maintained that 12 hours a day standing might be harmful for a child of six but not for a child of ten, for the "labour is so moderate it can scarcely be called labour at all". A Dr. Hardie said that the inhalation of cotton dust was not injurious "because the daily expectoration throws off the cotton and there is no accumulation in the lungs", while another medical witness was loath to admit that recreation and amusement were necessary for the development of healthy and happy young people. The Bill however was passed and a further step in factory legislation was taken.

A picture of child life at this time would not be complete without a reference to the meagre arrangements for any kind of religious or secular education then available for the majority of children, and the name of John Pounds (1766-1839), the cripple cobbler of Portsmouth, who attracted the neighbouring children into his dingy and ill-lit workshop and there strove to encourage them to master the three R's, should be mentioned. John Pounds and the workers of the London City Mission may be considered the real pioneers of Ragged Schools, which were established in 1835 and later were encouraged to great activity under their President, the Earl of Shaftesbury.

Beside the work of this pioneer reformer that of Thomas Cranfield (1766-1838) must be placed, for in 1798 he began to work among the slum children in Southwark, London, his efforts being directed towards the founding of a Sunday School for slum children who were too ragged and verminous to attend the more respectable Sunday Schools and Ragged Schools in the district.

Shocked by prevailing conditions, the writers of the day showed clearly that a humanitarianism was stirring in the heart of the country and Elizabeth Barrett Browning, Charles Blake and Thomas Hood brought to light, with poetic appeal, the hardships under which women and children were labouring in industry. The following are extracts from their poems:

" The Cry of the Children"—Elizabeth Barrett Browning (1844).

> Do you hear the children weeping, O my brothers,
>   Ere the sorrow comes with years?
> They are leaning their young heads against their mothers,
>   And that cannot stop their tears.
>
> The young lambs are bleating in the meadows,
>   The young birds are chirping in the nest,
> The young fawns are playing with the shadows,
>   The young flowers are blowing toward the west—
> But the young, young children, O my brothers,
>   They are weeping bitterly!
> They are weeping in the playtimes of the others,
>   In the country of the free.

" The Chimney Sweeper "—from *Songs of Innocence*. Charles
Blake (1789-1794).

> When my mother died I was very young,
> And my father sold me while yet my tongue
> Could scarcely cry weep! weep! weep! weep!
> So your chimneys I sweep, and in soot I sleep.

" The Song of the Shirt "—Thomas Hood (1843).

> With fingers weary and worn,
>> With eyelids heavy and red,
> A woman sat, in unwomanly rags,
> Plying her needle and thread—
>> Stitch! Stitch! Stitch!
> In poverty, hunger and dirt,
> And still with a voice of dolorous pitch
>> She sang the " Song of the Shirt ".

The prevailing industrial conditions at the time also inspired
a flood of novels. Mrs. Frances Trollope published *Michael
Armstrong, The Factory Boy* in 1840. This was followed by
Disraeli's *Sybil* and Mrs. Gaskell's *Mary Barton* and *North and
South*. Elizabeth Gaskell, the wife of a Unitarian Minister in
Manchester, had every opportunity for studying the daily
social problems of the mill girls she championed. In *Mary
Barton* her denunciation of the day-dreaming mentality which
made so many of them escape in phantasy from their class
only to drift into a life of prostitution proved her to have
been their warm-hearted friend. Charles Kingsley's *Yeast*
(1848), *Alton Locke* (1850), Charlotte Brontë's *Shirley* (1849),
Dickens's *Hard Times* (1854) all enrich the literature of the age,
each novelist taking the new industrial age as an absorbing
theme.

Medical literature also was appearing on the subject and in
1831 Charles Turner Thackrah, M.D., of Leeds, published *The
Effects of The Principal Arts, Trades and Professions on Health*.
Although this appeared about 132 years after Ramazzini's work
the content of both books is strikingly similiar. In the foreword
to Thackrah's book it is laid down that " a study of medicine

which disregards the prevention of disease, limits its ability and honours ". As stated in the sub-title the book deals with *The Effects of Arts, Trades and Professions and of Civic States and Habits of Living on Health and Longevity with suggestions for the removal of many of the agents which produce disease and shorten the duration of life.*

Thackrah quotes a paragraph from a contemporary report of the Manchester Board of Health as follows: " They have still to lament the untimely and protracted labour of children employed in some of the mills which tends to diminish future expectations as to the general sum of life and industry, by impairing the strength and destroying the vital stamina of the rising generation. At the same time it gives encouragement to idleness, extravagance and profligacy in the parents who, perverting the order of nature, subsist by the oppression of their offspring."

Among the industries fully described by Thackrah from his study in Leeds where industry took a toll of 450 people a year are the following: agricultural labourers, bakers, chimney sweeps, dressmakers, file cutters, hatters, iron miners, literary men, pearl button makers, scourers of wool, straw bonnet makers and worsted spinners, etc.

A murmuring from thoughtful men and women and the public generally grew in intensity and soon began to draw attention to the evil effects of child labour. The results of long hours, bad conditions and industrial hazards were clearly indicated by an increase in rickets and other physical deformities and from Bradford it is recorded that a woollen manufacturer complained to a Leeds surgeon that his mill children were being crippled by long hours and bad factory conditions.

In fairness to industry it must not be thought that the new era was responsible for all the misery of the day. In 1832 it is known that 50,000 souls died in the cholera epidemic; open sewers ran through the London streets; rows of back-to-back houses were built in the industrial districts and a supply of clean water was the privilege of a few. The infant mortality rate was over 150 per 1,000 live births.

At last, however, the Government of the country was aroused to action and in 1833 a Factories Enquiry Commission was set up. Sir Michael Sadler, Tory M.P. for Newark, was Chairman. The terms of reference were " To collect information in the manufacturing districts with respect to the employment of children in factories and to devise the best means for the curtailment of their labour." The members of the Commission were Thomas Tooke, an economist, Edwin Chadwick, a Poor Law Commissioner and public health reformer, and Southwood Smith, a housing reformer. The industrial country was divided into four parts and to each two civil commissioners and one medical commissioner were sent. At first the Commission was met with hostility because its sessions were held in secret and no evidence was taken from the children. It is recorded that conflicting evidence was given, some doctors being bribed to say it was even beneficial for the children's health to work long hours. A survey was made of 200 families in Bradford many members of which were deformed and were brought to the Commission to demonstrate the unnatural movements necessary in their work which had caused their disability.

When the Commission visited Leeds *The Times* of May 22, 1833, gave an amusing description of their reception. They were besieged by a mob of 3,000 singing children who surrounded the Town Hall and lustily made their opinions known, the burden of their song being:

> " We will have the ten hours bill
>   That we will, that we will.
> Else the land shall ne'er be still,
> Never still, never still.
> Parliament say what you will
>   We want no commissioning
> We will have the ten hour bill
>   That we will, that we will."

The petition, the words of which are attributed to Richard Oastler, known as the Factory Children's King, reads: " We protest against this commission as being founded on injustice, inhumanity and fraud to the interests of those who seek to continue slavery and its attendant ills ".

Two interesting resolutions passed at a public meeting in Huddersfield also show the rising anger against child labour. They ran as follows: " We are at loss for words to express our disgust and indignation at having been threatened with a visit from an inquisitorial itinerant to enquire whether our children shall be worked more than 10 hours a day. We are once and for all determined that they shall not." Also " That the present factory system can no longer be endured, that the evils it does inflict are unspeakably grievous to the working classes and their children and that the enemies of the poor have added treason and insult and injury by abusing the prerogative of the Crown and appointing a set of worthless Commissioners to perpetuate infant murder."

The Commission worked swiftly and reported as follows: " That excessive fatigue, privation of sleep, pain in the body, swelling of the feet, coupled with constant standing, the peculiar attitudes of the body, the peculiar motions of the limbs required in the labour of the factory, together with the elevated temperature and impure atmosphere do sometimes, ultimately, terminate in the production of serious permanent and incurable diseases, appears to us to be established." An outburst of disapproval from industrial members of parliament followed and William Cobbett in debate in the House said: " At one time it was said that the Navy was the great support of England; at another her maritime commerce and another her Colonies and another her Bank. Now it seems our great bulwark is 30,000 little mill girls ! "

Parliament took immediate action and in that same year the first Factory Act, a Whig Government measure, described as an " Act to regulate the labour of children and young persons in mills and factories ", was passed. It covered cotton, woollen, worsted, flax and silk mills.

The Act required:

1. The appointment of 4 inspectors, to cover the 3,000 existing factories. These men were Leonard Horner, Thomas Jones Howell, Robert Rickards and Robert Jones Saunders. They replaced the visitors under the 1802 Act and could impose penalties on the spot. Their salary was £1,000 a year.

2. The minimum age of employment was to be 9 years—no person under 18 to work more than ten hours a day—no person under 21 to work at night.

3. From 9-13 children were to attend school 12 hours a week.

4. It laid on industry the responsibility of establishing day schools. Horner, one of the Inspectors, a most unusual man, used interesting methods in his work. He called employers together in conference to explain the Act to them. He appealed to the humanitarian side of their natures and asked for co-operation and understanding in carrying out the law.

5. Children aged 9-13 years were not to be employed in any factory without a certificate from a surgeon of their physical ability.

The practical enforcement of this Act was fraught with difficulty. It must be remembered there was no compulsory registration of births until 1837 so the Factory Inspectors spent much of their time finding out the ages of the boys and girls at work. The practice whereby parents gave gin to their children to keep them small so they would be employed in the mills was now replaced by giving them an infusion of indigo which had the effect of making them look older than their tender years. This Act required a certificate to establish age, but if this was not procurable a child of four feet three and half inches in height was passed for employment.

But the first step had been taken. Horner, one of the first inspectors, encouraged employers to establish libraries and schools. He was responsible for 20 schools being started in Wigan and it is said one of his first duties was to dismiss a schoolmaster because he was unable to write. He held conferences with the millowners and by persuasion and education brought about many reforms.

According to the early reports of the factory inspectors, which make interesting reading, it seems to have been rather a point of honour that the firm should look after people who had been injured in their service. At this same time the reports of factory inspectors were filled with accounts of relief work and measures taken to produce occupation and instruction during periods of trade depression. Mr. Baker, an Inspector, reports: " It has been a source of gratification to me to find Mr. Sub-Inspector May, assisted by Mrs. May, instituting a night school for factory operatives during the long leisure of their bad time." This refers to the cotton famine in Lancashire due to the American Civil War when 43 per cent of operatives in Lancashire were out of work and 30 per cent on short time.

In England education figures largely in all early welfare schemes because there was no free education until 1870, and it is a tribute to industry that some of the first schools were established by employers in the early factories. It must also be remembered that the new industrialists were regarded as an inferior class by the old land-owning and merchant families, and they were also cut off from the culture of the ruling classes by the fact that most of them were Nonconformists. Being debarred from the universities they had to provide their own education and could adapt it to the needs of the time. Hence the Nonconformist academies were the most advanced educational establishments in eighteenth-century England. No wonder then that the provision of schools for the young factory " hands " was one of the earliest " welfare " activities in industry.

But it must not be thought there were no bright spots in Industrial England. As early as 1812 it is recorded that an eminent worsted spinner in Bradford employed a doctor at his mill and sent his ill and deformed children for treatment in

Derbyshire. This employer, named Wood, and his collaborator, Walker, had already established a ten-hour day for their children. They set up schools where needlework and other domestic subjects were taught. At North Shore Mill, Old Swann, Liverpool, where 850 workers, 52 per cent of whom were children, were employed, there was a complete health service in operation. Dr. W. T. Callan was the certifying surgeon in the district and the details of the service which are on record are interesting, showing the early trends of industrial welfare. For the salary of £200 a year a doctor attended at the surgery daily from 12-1 p.m. He distributed the hospital tickets. The employees contributed 1d. a week towards the expenses of the service. At this factory 200 children received daily instruction and there was night school from 8-9 p.m. A high sense of religious duty also influenced this welfare service, and religious instruction and compulsory attendance at Church and Sunday School were general. Additional amenities included a lending library, brass band, savings bank, New Year supper, annual picnic, and sick relief fund to which fines for misdemeanours were given. A messroom was also provided.

It is also recorded to the credit of a Liverpool factory that "Festive Meetings" were regularly held, for "in the month of July, the anniversary of the establishment of the Sunday School is celebrated by an excursion to the other side of the river originally confined to the children attending the School only but now extending to all those persons employed in the Mill whose general good conduct entitled them to a ticket upon their being able to give satisfactory proof of being in the habit of attending some place of instruction or public worship on the Sunday." The number varied from 600 to 700. Two steamboats were chartered for the occasion and an adequate supply of sandwiches and currant loaves taken; all the requisites for making and distributing coffee on the ground were available and the day was spent with hilarity in the fields on the Cheshire shore. It was said that "looking forward to this annual event acts well as a stimulus to good conduct and to a better observance of the Sabbath Day."

Little is known about conditions in the distributive trades at this time but a description of a general store in 1854 tells amusingly of life among the living-in shop apprentices of that day. The following rules were laid down for employees and clerks. " Store must not be opened on the Sabbath Day unless absolutely necessary and then only for a few minutes." " Any employee who is in the habit of smoking Spanish cigars, getting shaved at a barber's shop, going to dances and other such places of amusement, will most surely give his employer reason to be suspicious of his integrity and all round honesty." " Each employee must pay not less than one guinea per year to the Church and must attend Sunday School every Sunday." " Men employees are given one evening a week for courting purposes and two if they go to a prayer meeting regularly." " After 14 hours' work in the store the leisure time must be spent in reading good literature."

The mining industry also received some kindly consideration for there are records showing how Lady Bassett, acting on the suggestion of Dr. Carlyon, practising near the Dalcoath tin mine in Cornwall, arranged that the miners, instead of coming out on to the bleak hillside and drinking beer in a shed, could have provided for them, warm drying rooms, with baths and hot water supplied from the steam furnace. At this same mine hot pea soup instead of beer was served in another room.

Edwin Chadwick also mentions in his *Report on an enquiry into the sanitary conditions of the labouring population in Great Britain*, published in 1842, that Mr. James Smith of Deanston, near Stirling, retained the services of a medical gentleman to inspect the workpeople from time to time and give them timely advice and as far as possible to prevent disease.

Any discussion of prevailing conditions in this period would be incomplete without reference to one of the greatest industrial reformers of that age. Robert Owen is often quoted as saying: "We manufacturers are always perfecting our dead machinery, but of living machinery we are taking no care ", though his remarks must be directed to others rather than to the pioneer himself. Owen was born in 1771 and was the son of an ironmonger in a small town in North Wales. He was at the age of ten apprenticed to a draper but his ambitions quickly encouraged him to set up his own cotton mills in New Lanark. He was a man of character, almost a century before his time in thought and understanding. He refused to employ children under ten years of age; he built decent houses and schools which had a world-wide reputation. His employees were paid higher wages and worked shorter hours than in the neighbouring mills. His philosophy was described as the New Socialism and in practice many services not yet general in industry today were experiments at New Lanark. Such a man naturally inspired men of similiar thought and aspirations and the names of Richard Oastler, John Fielden, an eminent master spinner at Todmorden, Wood and Walker of Bradford, the Rev. J. R. Stephens, a Methodist preacher, and William Wilberforce come to mind. All entered the arena in their different spheres of influence to free not only the slaves in the West Indies for which Wilberforce worked so long, but the child slaves in the industrial North, and a long battle was about to begin.

The Earl of Shaftesbury.

Sir Michael Sadler, who headed the Factories Enquiry Commission, was not returned as a member in the Reform Parliament in 1832. Lord Ashley, later to become the seventh Earl of Shaftesbury, was therefore asked to accept leadership in a campaign still directed against the persistent evils of child labour. His benevolent interest in the little boy sweeps had been recognised when he was offered, and accepted, the Presidency of the " Climbing Boys Society ". This was a

Society of Members of Parliament who worked long and steadily for the abolition of a practice which can only be described as a blot on the happiness of child life in England. Realising the shortcomings of the Sadler Commission, which took no evidence from the factory children, Shaftesbury succeeded in persuading the Government to set up another committee and as a result a modest act applying to children in the cotton mills only was put upon the statute book. It not only forbade the employment of children under 9 years but also limited the hours from 9-16 years to 12 a day. There were, however, no arrangements for inspection and so the Act was soon a dead letter, it being looked upon as a tool of the employers rather than a protection for the children.

Shaftesbury continued the campaign both in and out of Parliament, never swerving from his main purpose. His writings and his bitter speeches, inspired by a deep religious fervour, slowly but surely wore down the opposition. His sincerity, evidenced by his practical interest in the Ragged School movement, the establishment of Sunday Schools and other humanitarian objects, endeared him to the people's hearts. The beauty of Eros in Piccadilly Circus, erected by money largely subscribed by the people he had lived to help, is a constant reminder of the great love and affection shown to him.

Shaftesbury knew his facts and marshalled them in speeches which remain classics today. An extract dealing with one aspect of child exploitation may be quoted as an illustration:

In the House he is reported to have said:

"To foster a supply of child labour in pin factories, masters resorted to the custom of lending money to parents on the credit of their children's toil; with the result that hapless youngsters became legally bound to pay off their parent's debt. Hence for drunken, degenerate parents the temptation of money in advance was too great to be resisted; and so the custom flourished."

Opposition, however, died slowly and many of the great

industrial Members of Parliament led by John Bright were vociferous in their condemnation of Shaftesbury's efforts. He resigned his seat in the Corn Law repeal agitation and John Fielden, member for Oldham, a cotton manufacturer, took charge of the 10-hour Bill, which was not, however, passed until 1847. By this Act hours for women and young persons were limited to ten and must be worked between 6 a.m. and 6 p.m. But the battle was not won, for the employers saw loopholes in the legislation and for their own advantage arranged a system of relays and shifts, defeating in some measure the main objects of the legislation. Shaftesbury saw the evils of child labour in spheres other than manufacturing and as a result of the second report of the Children's Employment Commission many reforms were made. For instance in the Calico Print Works some children began labour at 3-4 years, working 14-16 hours consecutively in a temperature of 100°, the air fouled by dust and chemicals. One more victory however was won when in 1845 the Print Works Act was passed by which no child under 8 could be employed in these works. Other clauses in the Act laid down that women and children must not work at night, all under 13 must attend school at least 30 days in each half year, exclusive of Sundays, and all Print Works must be inspected.

Other horrors were brought to light which resulted in the passing of the Agricultural Gangs Act. Brutal gang masters employed small children for work in the fields and as they usually contracted with a farmer it was to the master's interest to squeeze the maximum of labour from each child. Edwin Hodder in his *Life of Shaftesbury* gives a vivid description of their lot, " Year in, year out, in summer heat and winter cold; in sickness and in health with backs warped and aching from constant stooping; with hands blistered from pulling turnips and fingers lacerated from weeding among the stones; these English slaves, with education neglected, with morals corrupted, degraded and brutalised, labour from early morning till late at night and by the loss of all things gain the miserable pittance that barely keeps them from starvation."

The Agricultural Gangs Act of 1865 required:

1. No female under 18 to be employed in any public gang.
2. No child under 8 to be employed for hire in field labour of any sort.
3. No child between 8-13 to be employed for hire without producing a satisfactory certificate of school attendance.

Laws are always notorious for their loopholes and in spite of the amended Factory Acts of 1864 and 1867 by which all women, children and young persons were protected by legislation it was found that, technically, brickyard children were still outside the scope of all these measures. Carrying heavy loads of bricks distances up to 14 miles a day for long hours and under appalling conditions was a burden on child life which once more aroused Shaftesbury's wrath and his agitation led to further legislation in 1872 known as the Factory Acts (Bricks and Tile Yards) Extension Act.

As long ago as 1785 *A Sentimental History of the Chimney Sweepers in London and Westminster* was published by another philanthropist, Jonas Hanway, who was also the inventor of the umbrella. He drew attention to the miserable condition of boy sweeps and, due in large measure to the work of Shaftesbury when President of the Climbing Boys Society, an Act of 1834 ordered that flues, unless they were circular measuring 12 inches in diameter, were to measure 14 inches by 9 inches so that the danger of suffocation should be diminished. It also forbade a master sweep to employ a child under 10 years. Not until 1875, however, was there adequate legislation which then required master sweeps to hold a licence to employ boy sweeps which must be renewed annually by the police. The supply of boy sweeps was recruited in much the same way as for the cotton mills, but the suffering of the small boys was even greater. In *Oliver Twist*, that villainous master sweep Camfield will be remembered. Replying to the question " I

suppose he's fond of chimney sweeping?" Bumble remarked
"He dotes on it, your Worship!" A contribution in literature
to this campaign is the delightful story of *The Water Babies*,
expressly written in 1863 by Charles Kingsley to arouse public
opinion against one more black spot in child life.

No field of exploitation escaped Shaftesbury's penetrating
investigation and the employment of women and children in
the coal mines aroused his most vehement opposition and
unabated effort. A quotation from one of his speeches in the
House shows his deep concern over the abuses from which
the women had no escape. He said in 1842:

"The toil of females has hitherto been considered the characteristic of savage life; but we, in the height of our refinement,
impose on the wives and daughters of England a burden from
which, at least during pregnancy, they would be excepted in
slave-holding states, and among the Indians of America. . . .
But every consideration sinks to nothing compared with that
which springs from the contemplation of the moral mischiefs
this system engenders and sustains. You are poisoning the very
sources of order and happiness and virtue . . . you are annulling,
as it were, the institution of domestic life decreed by Providence
himself, the wisest and kindest of earthly ordinances, the mainstay
of social peace and virtue, and therein of national security. There
is a time to be born, and a time to die—this we readily concede;
but is there not also a time to live, to live to every conjugal and
parental duty?—this we seem as stiffly to deny . . . Sir, these
sources of mischief must be dried up; every public consideration
demands such an issue, the health of females, the care of their
families, their conjugal and parental duties, the comfort of their
homes, the decency of their lives, the rights of their husbands,
the peace of society and the laws of God; and until a vote shall
have been given this night—which God avert—I never will
believe that there can be found in this House one individual man
who will deliberately and conscientiously inflict on the women
of England such a burden of insufferable toil."

Shaftesbury pressed for a Royal Commission, which was soon
at work.

At the same time Sir Seymour Tremenheere, an Inspector

of Mines, submitted official reports which corroborated the evidence from all other sources and in 1842 a Mines Act was passed forbidding the employment of women and girls underground, the age limit for boys being 10.

To a citizen of the City of Gloucester may be given the credit of founding the first Sunday School. Robert Raikes, son of Robert Raikes the Elder, was born in 1736 and on the death of his father inherited the *Gloucester Journal*, of which he was both printer and editor. This newspaper was a medium through which Raikes persistently drew attention to the social problems of the day. It maintained (and still does) a high standard of journalism and the side of the downtrodden or unfortunate has always been put forward through its columns. Raikes first turned his practical attention to the sordid condition of the prisoners in Gloucester's two gaols. Infection was rampant but he showed no fear and visited the cells, where he would read aloud to the prisoners. Sometimes he would take the Bible as his subject but he was always anxious to introduce news from the outside world to bring an interest to the inmates. The story is told that the inspiration to bring children together on Sunday for religious instruction came from a chance remark of a Gloucester woman. He was looking at a gang of wild children playing in the streets. Their language was bad and they showed little control or discipline. He spoke to a woman who said, "You should come here on a Sunday when there are more children at play. The pin factories are closed that day and the children have nothing to do. It is hell let loose." Gloucester had long been the centre of the pin industry. "Parish apprentices" were employed in the same way as in the wool and cotton mills in the North. Hours were incredibly long and the influence of home life was unknown, for the children were generally orphans and laboured under conditions of slavery. Their work was monotonous and only little fingers could stick the rows of pins so regularly in the long sheets of paper, in which pins were arranged for sale until recently.

Raikes believed that idleness bred lawlessness and his plan to collect the children on Sundays met with a ready response. The school hours were from 8 a.m. to 11 a.m. followed by a church service. They returned at 2 o'clock and worked till 6 p.m.

The curriculum was simple as few children could read. Often the Bible was the textbook. Raikes was loved by the children and slowly but surely a change came over the town and employers recognised a good influence was abroad. After three years of experiment Raikes published, through the *Gloucester Journal*, an account of his work. The idea spread rapidly and from so humble a beginning a great nation-wide educational system has sprung.

Royal interest was also shown in Gloucester's pin industry when Queen Charlotte, the Queen of George III, visited the pin factory of Messrs. Weaver. The Court had moved to Cheltenham in 1788 for the King to " take the waters " and the Queen showed a deep interest in the social improvements that were taking place in Gloucester. On her return to Windsor she asked Robert Raikes to see her, and Sunday Schools were established there soon after his visit.

In another direction, during this period, the vigorous religious preaching throughout the length and breadth of the country of John Wesley and George Whitefield aroused the dulled conscience of the people. There emerged a flood of Methodism radiating a spiritual influence over the country, which, passing through economic and social changes of such great magnitude, needed spiritual guidance and support in its great endeavours.

As a background to this chapter of history some other contemporary happenings during the struggle against child labour can be cited, indicative of the general yearning among men for a better life, for freedom from oppression and for action to be taken against " man's inhumanity to man ". Soon after the abolition of slavery throughout the British Empire in 1833 came the banishment of the Tolpuddle martyrs to Botany Bay. The Registration of Births Act in 1837 and the accession of Queen Victoria in the same year preceded the Education Act of 1839. Not until 1847 was the 10-hour Act finally passed and the following year the first great Public Health Act was put on the Statute Book. In this year it may be recalled that Sir John Simon was appointed as the first Medical Officer of Health. It was largely due to the efforts of Sir Edwin Chadwick, the great public health and social reformer, through his comprehensive surveys of the low health standards of the country, that the need for such an appointment was brought to the notice of the Government. In 1855 a Medical Officer was employed by W. H. Smith & Son Ltd., Dr. Jenner had already developed his theory of vaccination against smallpox, and Pasteur published his first research findings on alcoholic fermentation in 1857.

The Crimean War is essentially a landmark in any review of nursing history and the work of Florence Nightingale must be mentioned as the herald of a new era in the development of public health nursing in this country. Although Florence Nightingale cannot be claimed as having made a direct contribution to industrial nursing, yet from her writings, and particularly *Notes on Nursing* published in 1859, her influence was so widespread, penetrating all levels of thought from the Cabinet to more humble citizens, that its extent can never be estimated. Acting on her advice the Ladies' Sanitary Reform Society of Manchester began a health visiting and infant welfare service. Buckingham County Council much later employed Health Missioners and Florence Nightingale's comment when advising Sir Frederick W. Verney, Chairman, North Buckinghamshire Technical Education Committee, on the appointment of these health workers in 1892 was to the effect that the necessary stock in trade of anyone who wants to be a health missioner is " some knowledge and much sympathy ". At the same time in relation to the development of rural health work in Buckinghamshire, she says: "The only word that sticks is the word that follows work." And in a message to the first recruits in this pioneer health service she says: "The work that pays is the work of the skilful hand directed by the cool head and inspired by the loving heart. Join heart with heart and hand in hand and pray for the perfect gift of love to be the spirit and life of all your work." Whilst there is no definite evidence that in those early days Florence Nightingale influenced the development of industrial nursing specifically, yet one of her prophetic utterances surely inspires all industrial nursing today. She said: "Nursing is not only a service to the sick—it is a service also to the well—we have to teach people how to live." As a direct result of Miss Nightingale's influence William Rathbone of Liverpool started a district nursing service in that city in 1859. The same year Henri Dunant founded the Red Cross after the battle of Solferino.

In other spheres of public service many awakenings of the social conscience were becoming apparent and the names of eminent men and women are woven into the tapestry of voluntary social work during this period of rapid growth towards a humanising of the social structure of the country. Elizabeth Fry, for her work among women prisoners in Newgate Gaol, and Octavia Hill, in the realms of housing and education, stand on the hilltop of reform, and the Invalid Children's Aid Association soon developed as a result of the pressing need discovered by the latter. For her educational work among the lawless and primitive people living isolated in the Mendip Hills, the name of Hannah More is remembered. In 1869 Charles Stewart Loch founded the Charity Organisation Society—now the Family Welfare Association—and Benjamin Waugh laid the foundation on which was built the National Society for the Prevention of Cruelty to Children. In another sphere Seebohm Rowntree was drawing public attention to facts about poverty and its consequences which he published in statistical surveys, and Beatrice and Sidney Webb contributed their *Fabian Essays on Socialism* to the literature on this subject. The principles underlying the establishment of community settlements has been outlined by Canon Bartlett, the founder of Toynbee Hall, and in 1883 the Women's Co-operative Guild commenced to work towards a more enlightened outlook for women on the evils of the day. This period was overflowing with inspiration from the fertile minds of men and women in all walks of life and much of it led to positive action reflected in the many movements which influence social life today.

3

Industrial Nursing is Born

It was against this grim background of industrial life that the deepening humanitarianism so characteristic of the middle of the nineteenth century was reflected, and the first industrial nurse comes into the picture. This story of her discovery is a romantic episode.

It was in 1937 that the International Council of Nurses was meeting in Congress in London and the writer was asked to read a paper on " Industrial Nursing in Great Britain ". Up to this time the Vermont Marble Company in the United States of America was given in the textbooks as the first company to employ industrial nurses, but it was thought that the earlier industrialisation of England suggested an earlier industrial nursing development. In order to establish this fact wide inquiries were made, many directed to the Quaker firms. It was known that J. S. Fry & Sons, Ltd., Bristol; Cadbury Bros., Ltd., Birmingham; Reckitt & Sons, Hull; J. &. J. Colman, Norwich; C. & J. Clark Ltd., Street, Somerset; and Mardon, Son & Hall, Bristol, had early been in the field of industrial welfare and had already established extensive health and educational activities of many kinds but no dates were available when a nurse was first employed. The inquiry aroused interest and minute books were taken down from their dusty shelves in factory offices in a search for the necessary evidence. But nothing was forthcoming.

An approach to the late Miss Ethel and the late Miss Helen Colman of Carrow Abbey, Norwich, however, ultimately proved fruitful. As little girls they remembered a nurse coming to their home. They made exhaustive enquiries in Norwich and the "oldest inhabitants" interviewed also remembered a nurse when they were boys in the mustard factory of J. & J. Colman. But no name or date could be given. The life and work of Mrs. J. J. Colman, their mother, is well known. She came of a Puritan family and married James Colman of Stoke Holy Cross. Inspired by a deep desire to help her husband's workpeople she formed in 1872 the Carrow Works Self Help Medical Club, the object of which was " to enable the wives and families of men employed at the Carrow Works to obtain efficient medical attendance by the payment of a small monthly subscription ". A doctor attended at the works dispensary on Mondays and Wednesdays at 11 a.m. and on Fridays at 10 a.m. Mrs. Colman also established schools where the curriculum, including Venetian iron work, cookery, bee-keeping, gardening, laundry, and embroidery, showed how modern was her conception of education. She arranged for Sunday Schools as part of the community service, taking the senior girls' class herself, and soup kitchens were directed under her personal supervision. In 1874 it was recorded that Mrs. Colman appointed Miss Kate Southall, a welfare worker, whose duties were mainly among the girls and women employees.

In the spring of 1937 Miss Helen Colman, though still continuing her search, feared the necessary information would remain sunk in oblivion. But in spring-cleaning a cupboard in her mother's bedroom a bundle of small flimsy-leaved notebooks was discovered where cash payments and the results of the yearly examinations at Carrow School were entered. The ink was faded and hardly decipherable. The entries were in shorthand, a style now obsolete but used among the Colman family to communicate with each other. Always bearing in mind her quest Miss Colman read through the little books and found the following entry, which she alone could transcribe: " Philippa Flowerday aged 32, engaged October 1878 at 26s. a week, on condition of her father's moving to live near Carrow as soon as he can find a suitable cottage." In another book was an entry confirming this. It read " Philippa Flowerday aged 32, engaged October 1878 at 26s. a week as district nurse."

Very little is known of this pioneer industrial nurse, but a few details were given later by Miss Emily Quarry who succeeded her at Carrow Works in 1888 when Philippa left to be married to the Colman gardener and became Mrs. William Reid. From Miss Quarry, an old lady of over 90 when she was visited in hospital, it was learned that Philippa Flowerday was trained at the Norfolk and Norwich Hospital, although this cannot be confirmed as records were not kept until much later. However, in a report of the Board in 1875 it says that pyaemia and erysipelas had continued to occur in the wards during portions of the year and the committee strongly recommended the improvement of the hospital nursing arrangements and the formation of a training school and home for nurses in connection with the hospital under the general charge of the Lady Superintendent who must herself be a trained nurse. This recommendation was adopted and a Miss Graham was appointed the first Lady Superintendent and head of the nurses at a salary of £100 a year. Dr. Beverley of Norwich was surgeon to the hospital at that time and it is owing to his memory that it can be confirmed that Philippa Flowerday was at the hospital, because he remembered her and produced for Miss Colman a group picture in which she appears with her colleagues.

An interesting letter from Mrs. Colman to her husband records her method of approach when the idea of a nurse for the factory came first to her mind. She says, "I strongly feel that Miss Southall is doing a *great deal* of good in a quiet way among the girls by showing them how willing she is to take any trouble if she can but teach them to be better women and better wives as they grow up, and I have been thinking that there is an immense amount of work to be done especially now that the girls are beginning to buy calico and flannel and want to be taught how to make it up." This letter was preparatory to a request for more help which Jeremiah Colman and his partners were willing to supply. Miss Southall had been appointed to work among the factory girls, one of her duties being to conduct sewing classes.

When Philippa Flowerday was appointed she was already employed by the Norwich Staff of Nurses with headquarters at Bethel Street, Norwich, which later became the Norwich District Nursing Association, at one time housed at the Cavell Home in Tombland, and it is no wonder therefore that she interpreted her work on district nursing principles. It is known that she reported on duty at Carrow factory at 9 a.m. working with the doctor till 11 a.m. Then, filling a large basket with good things from the Colman kitchen she spent the rest of the day tending the sick employees and their families in their own homes. Her average weekly visits were 45 and Mrs. Colman inspected her record book. She distributed Christmas parcels of blankets and other comforts and co-operated closely with the sick benefit society which administered a clothing club and lending library.

These few known facts illustrate a lesson which Philippa Flowerday has taught and which is apt to be forgotten in these modern and highly organised days. By her work she linked the factory and the home, thus keeping continuity of nursing care and by following up the patient in his home she could provide for many of his needs and also those of his family. From the Colman heritage, therefore, a family of Free Churchmen—Baptists, came the inspiration of industrial nursing. Jeremiah Colman's work for the Reform Bill, emancipation of the West Indian Slaves, abolition of the Corn Laws, the British and Foreign Bible Society, the Baptist Missionary Society, the Adult School movement, and many other steps towards civil and religious liberty, were reflected in the wide plans for industrial improvement which he fostered at Carrow Works.

The House of Courtauld.

From *A History of Courtauld* by C. H. Ward-Jackson, a wealth of detail is available, showing the broad conception of " welfare " which the founders of the House of Courtauld introduced into their firm from the early days of the nineteenth century. Extracts from this book give an interesting description of the day nursery initiated by Mrs. Samuel Courtauld; she also encouraged the mill girls to dress in a style suitable to their surroundings.

A notice, dated 1860, the original of which is still in existence, was hung on the factory wall and reads as follows:

DRESS

October 9th 1860

IT is always a pleasure to us to see our work-people, and especially our comely young women, dressed NEAT and TIDY; nor should we, as has been already declared in a notice that has been put up at Bocking Mills, wish to interfere with the fashion of their dress, whatever it may be, so long as their dress does not interfere with their work, or with the work of those near them in our employ.

The present ugly fashion of HOOPS, or CRINOLINE, as it is called, is, however, quite unfitted for the work of our Factories. Among the Power Looms it is almost impossible, and highly dangerous; among the Winding and Drawing Engines it greatly impedes the free passage of Overseers, Wasters, etc., and it is inconvenient to all. At the Mill it is equally inconvenient, and still more mischievous, by bringing the dress against the Spindles, while also it sometimes becomes shockingly indecent when the young people are standing upon the Sliders.

FOR ALL THESE REASONS

We now request all our Hands, at all our Factories, to leave HOOPS and CRINOLINE at home when they come to the Factories to work; and to come dressed in a manner suitable for their work, and with as much BECOMING NEATNESS as they can.

And OVERSEERS at all the Floors are hereby charged to see that all the Hands coming to work are thus properly dressed for factory work—without Hoops or Crinoline of any sort; and Overseers will be held RESPONSIBLE to us for strict regard to this regulation.

LICKING BOBBINS

When a Bobbin is fastened off, it has been a common practice to touch the end with the tongue to smooth it down, and there is no harm in that.

But out of this practice has arisen another practice, both nasty and mischievous, of licking the Bobbins all over to make them weigh heavier.

And to put an end at once, and altogether, to this nasty and mischievous practice of Licking the Bobbins, we now make it

A RULE

Not to touch the Bobbins with the Tongue at all, and Overseers are hereby authorised to endorse this rule by Forfeits.

SAMUEL COURTAULD & CO.

Other references are made in this history showing the similarity of political thought shared by the Courtauld family and other industrial families who were the great yeoman of industry. The following is an example: it is known that in 1852 the firm fitted up a lodging house at Halstead for young girls, with an institute and a library and an evening school. They also employed a lady visitor " whose occupation it was to visit the homes of the workpeople and inculcate habits of cleanliness and to provide them with some comforts in the case of sickness."

It is thought this " lady visitor " was Mary Merryweather, the friend of Bessie Parkes, who was a life-long friend of Barbara Bodichon, who, together with Emily Davies, founded Girton College, Cambridge. Bessie Parkes was editor of the *Englishwoman's Journal*. In this she wrote stirring articles about the work of Florence Nightingale (a cousin of Barbara Bodichon), Miss Bosanquet, Dr. Elizabeth Blackwell and other pioneers in the women's movement.

At this time, in many Victoria drawing rooms, the plea was being made by a brave group of far-seeing women, for a greater realisation of the work women could do. The infant welfare services were calling for help; women were needed in hospitals, in reform schools and in the asylums. In particular Mary Merryweather emphasised the need that existed for educated women to take up social work in factories such as she was doing " in Mr. Courtauld's silk factory at Halstead in Essex ". Similiar work was done at Braintree and at Bocking. A day nursery was initiated by Mrs. Samuel Court-auld, for the convenience of the mothers who worked at the Halstead factory. The mothers took the children at 6 a.m. and brought them home at 6 p.m. Whilst the mothers were nursing their children they were allowed to leave their work and come to the nursery at 8.15 a.m., 11 a.m., 1.15 p.m., and 4 p.m. The charge made was 1s. 6d. per week.

Another important step to be mentioned in this historical survey was the establishment in 1887 of the Queen Victoria Institute which was a Diamond Jubilee gift to Her Majesty from the women of the country. The sum of £70,000 was subscribed and at her special request was used for the training and development of nursing in the homes of the people.

Up to this time the abolition of child labour had not materially affected the employment of women in industry and appalling conditions were still general in many districts. The match girls employed in an East End factory, resenting a levy by the firm of 1s. a head to erect in the district a statue of Mr. Gladstone, were becoming restless. Phossy jaw was taking its toll in human suffering: 14 hours a day for a meagre wage of 4s. 6d. to 8s. weekly were worked in dreadful conditions. Sweated labour by the whole family, including the old people and children in the nearby homes, was a black spot soon to arouse public opinion once more. Mrs. Annie Besant, editor of the *Link*, supported by Bernard Shaw and other Fabians, brought the match girls out on strike in 1888, this unheard of action shocking the employers in their board room isolation. The same year Charles Booth, a wealthy shipowner, published his *Survey of Conditions in the East End*, showing the squalid and horrible conditions under which the people lived.

The women chain-makers of Cradley Heath were also attracting attention and other sweated industries such as lace making in Nottingham, dress making in Mayfair, net making at Bridport, carpet making at Kidderminster, and thread making at Kilbirnie were under criticism. Conditions of work in the jute and flax trade in Dundee were also the subject of investigation. Emma Paterson, a working woman, was the first to draw attention to the opportunities available through organisation for improving the conditions of women in these sweated industries. She founded the Women's Protective and Provident League, later to become the Women's Trade Union League, with offices in a dreary alley off Shaftesbury Avenue, but her death in 1886 was a serious blow to progress. It remained, however, for Lady Dilke, the wife of Sir Charles Dilke, Liberal M.P. for the Forest of Dean, to follow in her steps and carry on the torch. In this work she was assisted by her niece, Gertrude Tuckwell, and her private secretary, May Abraham, later Mrs. H. J. Tennant. Other women in the van of the movement towards the emancipation of women were Margaret MacDonald, wife of the Rt. Hon. Ramsey MacDonald, Lilian M. Faithfull and Dorothea Beale, Principals of the Cheltenham Ladies' College, Frances Mary Buss, Margaret Macmillan, Ellen Wilkinson, Annie Besant, Margaret Bondfield, Louisa Martindale and A. B. Barwell, Headmistress of the Girls' High School, Gloucester, Baroness Burdett Coutts, Emily Davies, Annie Kenney and Christabel Pankhurst. In a short history of this kind it is not possible to describe all the strong influences which were stirring in the struggle for emancipation of Victorian womanhood at this time, though the agitation so nobly fired by Josephine Butler against the Contagious Diseases Acts, disclosing the cruelty of commercialised vice to child victims,

must not remain unmentioned. Moreover the work of Millicent Fawcett for Women Suffrage and Elizabeth Garratt
Anderson for recognition of women in the medical field, is
an everlasting testimony of the tenacity of purpose of these
great pioneers.

But the outstanding figure in the struggle for better conditions of employment for women was Mary Macarthur.
Beginning as an active worker in the Shop Assistants' Union,
at the age of 23 she followed Lady Dilke as Secretary of the
Women's Trade Union League, a position for which she was
encouraged to apply by Margaret Bondfield and Gertrude
Tuckwell. This " slip of a girl, fair-headed, mounted on a
chair, speaking with great firmness and persuasiveness at a
factory gate ", rapidly became an outstanding figure not only
in trade union circles but in all progressive movements of
the country. One of the triumphs of this great woman was
the decision taken by the Government to investigate the
sweated industries. An exhibition of these industries was later
arranged in London and did much to arouse public opinion
against these injustices.

Side by side with the fearless work of Mary Macarthur,
important events were happening in the government supervision of factory conditions. In 1896 Arthur Whitelegge was
appointed Chief Inspector, Factory Department of the Home
Office, and was followed two years later by Dr. (later Sir)
Thomas Morison Legge as Chief Medical Officer, Factory
Department of the Home Office, whose outstanding researches
in toxicology have left a far-reaching effect on occupational
health. The Workmen's Compensation Act in 1906, the
Trade Boards Act introduced by Winston Churchill in 1909,
and the National Health Insurance Act and Old Age Pensions
by Lloyd George in 1911, built a firm foundation of social
services which were designed for the well-being of the industrial population, but the outbreak of war in 1914 intensified the
need for vigilance and careful planning of industrial legislation.

Returning to the work of Mary Macarthur, a survey of women in industry at this time describes the gigantic task before her. In 1914 there were just under 358,000 women in organised Unions, about two-thirds being in the textile trade. The right to speak for women munition workers who rallied to the call of their country when war was declared therefore had to be established.

Mary Agnes Hamilton in *Mary Macarthur—A Biographical Sketch*, describes how she was able to show, on the basis of an inquiry carried out by the National Federation of Women Workers, that the best ordinary rate for women was 15s. a week and the average much lower. There was no pretence of giving them equal rates with men. In fact, the employers, finding women efficient, defended the low rates they were paying by declaring that men had hitherto been paid too much. Alternatively they argued that they had had to introduce new machinery and that the women's wages ought to bear the cost of it.

The first Munitions Act (July 1915) did nothing to protect women. Some of its clauses, indeed, made their lot much worse. Thus, under the Act, strikes were forbidden, while Clause 7 (the famous Leaving Certificate Clause) made it practically impossible for a worker on any form of munitions to leave a job, no matter what the conditions or the pay.

Mary Macarthur put a simple point to Mr. Lloyd George: If you say to the women, " you are not to leave your employment," then you must make the conditions of that employment decent. In many cases women were regularly working between seventy and eighty hours a week, and this in factories and shops where there were no adequate sanitary or other arrangements for their comfort. These were the conditions to which they were chained by the Munitions Act, and for which they were being paid from 9s. to 15s. a week. At last, in September, 1915, her persistency compelled the appointment of a Committee of Inquiry.

The health question and the wages question were tied up together, and revelations about one helped to get action on the other. The Government set up the Labour Supply Committee in September 1915 and Mary Macarthur was a member. She had by now forced the position of women to the front and compelled her own recognition as their spokesman. She was never a mere member of any committee. The speed and efficiency with which this one got to business registers the effect of her drive.

A circular produced by the Committee contained a list of occupations suitable for women and urged the importance of providing lavatory and cloak-room accommodation for them. The Ministry of Munitions adopted these recommendations.

It was not until the appointment of the first four women inspectors in 1893, two to the Home Office and two to the Royal Borough of Kensington, that any progress was made in developing the idea of safeguarding the health of women working behind the machines. It is of particular interest to remember that two of the local inspectors, Miss Dean and Miss R. E. Squire, who were both later promoted to the Home Office, trained under the National Health Society with a view to qualifying as lecturers on Hygiene, Nursing and First Aid for that Society. Both these inspectors were probationers at the Chelsea Infirmary and later trained as district nurses with the Queen Victoria Jubilee Institute. They obtained the Diploma of the National Health Society in Anatomy, Physiology, Hygiene, Nursing and First Aid.

In her book *Thirty Years in the Public Service*, Miss Squires says, "such qualifications would be of themselves scarcely reckoned now sufficient to secure women an appointment to an important post but they were at least equal to those produced by our competitors. The training, in fact, proved to be exceedingly useful in the exercise of our duties both during our work under the sanitary authority and also afterwards when we went to the Home Office."

No history touching on the early efforts to improve factory life would be complete without mention of the outstanding work of Hilda Martindale, C.B.E., formerly of the Home Office and the Treasury. At the time she became a lady factory inspector in 1901, there were 32,000 children from 12 years of age employed on the half-time system; in addition many thousands of children of 13 years of age and young persons of over 14 years were employed full time for 60 hours a week and those working in their own homes on sweated trades could not be numbered. Her investigations into the conditions under which children worked in the employment of Court dressmakers in Mayfair, in the potteries and brickfields and the linen and woollen industries in Ireland were extensive. Furthermore, the high-class laundry work often carried out by religious communities, orphanages and Rescue Homes in Ireland, sometimes under primitive conditions, was the subject of her intensive and penetrating survey. Her unfailing efforts to improve conditions by persuasion and through education of employers on their legal responsibilities brought about far-reaching improvements in conditions of work. To illustrate the extremes to which employers at that time would sometimes go, it is interesting to note that the Industrial Law Committee, which was founded by Gertrude Tuckwell, was urgently needed to indemnify workers who had been dismissed for answering truthfully questions put to them by factory inspectors. Only gradually did the workers appreciate the efforts being made on their behalf.

Miss Martindale's work in the Midlands during the first world war among industries of wide variety and each with its particular hazard laid foundation on which later health and welfare reforms were built, and in the 1920s, when any special regulations for dangerous trades and welfare orders for certain industries were made, her wide knowledge of the trade in question considerably influenced the conditions which were subsequently laid down. She was particularly concerned with the framing of Welfare Orders for fruit preserving, herring curing, laundries, bakehouses and biscuit factories. These Orders required the provision of protective clothing, of accommodation for clothing, of a suitable messroom, of first-aid boxes, of a supply of drinking water, and of seating accommodation under certain circumstances, of the provision of an ambulance room with a trained nurse in charge. The success of so much of Miss Martindale's work was partly due to the dawning of a new understanding between masters and men which had been fostered by the Report of the Whitley Committee under the Chairmanship of Mr. J. H. Whitley, M.P., then speaker of the House of Commons; this recommended the establishment of National Industrial Councils to be representative of both employers and employees, through which wages and conditions of employment could be negotiated jointly. Another manifestation of this new co-operative spirit was the formation of the British Industrial Safety First Association, resulting from a meeting of employers and employees which was called by the Lord Mayor of London. The outstanding work of Miss Martindale will also be remembered in connection with the establishment of the Home Office Museum, now the Health and Welfare Museum, Horseferry Road, S.W.1, the planning and arrangement of which was her own personal achievement.

4

The First World War

THE development of industrial health work after the outbreak
of war in 1914 and the part played by nurses finds little space
in the meagre literature written on the subject at that time, but
in a report of the filling factory at Georgetown, Renfrewshire,
it is said, " A welfare assistant attached to the staff of the
medical department had charge of the home visiting section.
Owing to the difficulty of workers and their dependants
resident in the houses belonging to the factory receiving
necessary attention in an emergency, it was found advisable
to engage a district nurse for this work. The services of the
Township nurse Miss Isobella Horne were much appreciated."

When Lloyd George became Minister of Munitions of
War in 1915 and National Shell Factories, National Filling
Factories and National Projectile Factories came under his
direct control he knew all was not well with the industrial
life of the country. Manufacturers were concerned at the
insobriety of the people. Drunkenness was rife among men and
women and there were indications that this state of affairs was
having a serious effect on production in those industries which
were necessary for the successful conduct of the grim war
struggle. The principles of Lloyd George, as a Welshman and a
Nonconformist who had been schooled in the hard but
straight way of temperance and a simple evangelism, naturally
appealed to the thousands of Free Churchmen in the country
who, up to this time, had not given wholeheartedly their
moral support to the war effort. Led by Dr. J. H. Shakespeare,

the secretary of the Baptist Union, together with other free church denominations the Nonconformist conscience rebelled against the depravity of national life and through various Church organisations rallied to the challenge of the great war leader.

Lloyd George quickly recognised the need for an urgent and all-round improvement in conditions of labour and appointed in 1915 a strong Governmental Committee, the Health of Munition Workers Committee, to consider the health and welfare of munition workers. The Committee met under the chairmanship of Sir George Newman, Chief Medical Officer of the Board of Education, the terms of reference being " to consider and to advise on questions of industrial fatigue, hours of labour and other matters affecting the personal health and physical efficiency of workers in munitions workshops and factories."

The members of this Committee were:

Sir George Newman, K.C.B., M.D., F.R.C.P. (Chairman), Chief Medical Officer, Board of Education, Member of the Central Control Board (Liquor Traffic); Emeritus Lecturer in Preventive Medicine at St. Bartholomew's Hospital.
Sir Thomas Barlow, Bart., K.C.V.O., M.D., LL.D., F.R.S., Physician Extraordinary to H.M. the King; late President of the Royal College of Physicians.
Gerald Bellhouse, Esq., C.B.E., H.M. Deputy Chief Inspector of Factories, Home Office.
Professor A. E. Boycott, M.D., F.R.S., Director of Pathological Department, University College, London.
J. R. Clynes, Esq., M.P., Parliamentary Secretary to the Ministry of Food.
E. L. Collis, Esq., M.B., H.M. Medical Inspector of Factories, Home Office; Director of Health and Welfare, Ministry of Munitions.
Sir Walter M. Fletcher, K.B.E., M.D., Sc.D., F.R.S., F.R.C.P., Secretary to the Medical Research Committee, Fellow of Trinity College, Cambridge.
Leonard E. Hill, Esq., M.B., F.R.S., Director, Department of

Applied Physiology and Hygiene, Medical Research Committee;
Professor of Physiology, London Hospital Medical School.
Samuel Osborn, Esq., J.P., Managing Director, Clyde Steel
Works, Sheffield.
Miss R. E. Squire, O.B.E., H.M. Deputy Principal Lady In-
spector of Factories, Home Office.
Mrs. H. J. Tennant, C.H.
E. H. Pelham, Esq. (Secretary); Assistant Secretary, Board of
Education.

The following are extracts from the final Report of the
Committee dealing with Industrial Health and Efficiency
published in 1918:

MEANS OF PREVENTION

In the majority of factories some provision is made for the treatment of injuries, but inspection indicates that there is great and
urgent need of improvement, especially for treating minor
injuries. While one factory may possess a well-equipped surgery
with a trained nurse in charge, at another provision for treatment
may be wholly absent, or the surgical equipment may be represented by a soiled roll of some so-called " antiseptic " lint or
gauze, an open packet of absorbent wool, a few bandages, some
antiseptic lotion, or an unclean pair of scissors, all kept in a dusty
drawer. It is obvious that provision of equipment for first aid
is worse than useless unless it is properly kept and maintained.
What is required is an adequate though simple organisation which
provides (a) a local dressing station or aid post in each workplace
for minor injuries; and (b) a central dressing station or surgery for
more serious cases requiring continuous treatment. An Order
recently made by the Home Office under the Police, Factories,
etc. (Miscellaneous. Provisions) Acts, 1916, Section 7 requires
that in the case of blast furnaces, copper mills, iron mills, foundries
and metal works, a first-aid box shall be provided in the proportion of at least one to every 150 persons, and an ambulance
room wherever 500 or more persons are employed. Arrangements
should also be made for the immediate conveyance to hospital
of cases which cannot be treated on the spot.

LOCAL DRESSING STATION OR AID POST

In order to be effective under industrial conditions any form of
treatment for minor injuries must be extremely simple, easily

understood and readily applicable. Elaborate provisions for the treatment of minor injuries is less necessary, because of its unsuitability under factory conditions, and because in machine shops wounds are usually comparatively free from germs. Further, the treatment must be always and promptly available. The workman who sustains a slight injury while at work will often decline to surrender a quarter of an hour of time and earnings in going to and from a central surgery to have his wound dressed. Time is a consideration, and the exigencies of factory life do not allow of an elaborate procedure. The aid post may take the form of a cupboard or box containing first-aid materials, with brief, simple and clear instructions as to their use. The box should contain packets of sterilised dressings, a supply of iodine solution (alcoholic solution containing 2 per cent iodine), a bottle of " eye drops ", a pair of dressing scissors, some triangular bandages, safety pins, and a roll of plaster (1 inch wide). The sterilised dressings may suitably be of three sizes:

(a) Three dozen small size, for fingers, composed of a strip of gauze or lint 8 inches long and 1 inch wide, with narrow tape attached to one end. The tape should be rolled up inside the strip, which is then wrapped in a cover of ordinary nonabsorbent wool and the whole sterilised. In use the wool is first removed and the dressing unrolled round the injured finger, when the tape is disclosed ready for tying the dressing in position.

(b) One dozen medium size, for hands or feet, similiar to the above, but 18 inches long and 1½ inches wide; and

(c) One dozen large size, for which the ordinary field dressing may be taken as a pattern.

The aid post should be under the care of an officer, preferably the foreman or forewoman, trained in first-aid work. This officer should keep a note of every case dressed, and should be responsible for seeing that the box is kept stocked and in proper order. Ordinarily one such aid post should be provided in each workplace, but in large engineering shops several may be required.

CENTRAL DRESSING STATION OR SURGERY

The Central Dressing Station should be easily accessible and specially constructed or adapted for the purpose. The room or rooms should, in large factories, provide for a surgery, a rest room, and a storeroom and nurses' room. Where a surgery is used for workers of both sexes a second small room will be found advantageous. The walls should be covered with glazed tiles, enamelled iron sheets, or washable paint. The floor should be of smooth, hard, durable and impervious material; the natural and artificial lighting should be ample, hot and cold water should be laid on or be immediately available; the room should be warmed in winter. A glazed sink is needed, the waste pipe opening over the drain, and trapped outside the surgery. A footbath, preferably fixed and provided with hot and cold water, is desirable. The furniture should consist of a table, a couch, chairs and cupboards. The room should not contain a carpet, rugs, curtains, table cloth, window blinds or wall pictures. The keynote should be simplicity and cleanliness. The floor should be washed once a day with antiseptic fluid, and the walls at least once a week. The objects of the central dressing station being the treatment of more serious cases than can be dealt with at the aid post, and the re-dressing of cases of minor injuries, it is desirable that it should be properly equipped. It may also be convenient to use it for the medical examination of applicants for work.

The station must be in charge of a competent person with knowledge of ambulance work. Wherever possible a trained nurse should be on regular duty, ambulance assistants being selected from employees trained in first-aid work. Many large works now have a medical officer on the staff, who is responsible for the supervision of the surgery and available for serious cases before removal to hospital.

The equipment of the surgery will largely depend upon the character of the accommodation provided and the experience of the person in charge, but the following will generally be required:

i. stretchers, splints and strong bandages for major accidents.

ii. bandages and dressings for minor injuries (a stock should be kept to replenish the aid posts);

iii. a simple steriliser and necessary surgical instruments such as scissors, forceps and tourniquet; and

iv. simple lotions and drugs (with sufficient enamelled basins).

Where a medical officer is employed at the factory he should be provided with accommodation adjoining the central dressing station. The accommodation should ordinarily include a consulting room . . . (fitted with hot and cold water and a steriliser), a clerk's office and a waiting room. If arrangements are made for men and women to attend at different hours a separate waiting room will not ordinarily be required.

The following statement is of interest, as showing the arrangements made at a large National Filling Factory for dealing with cases of sickness and injury:

AMBULANCE EQUIPMENT. At each of two factories we have a roomy ambulance building with accommodation for doctor's consultations, first-aid dressings, sickness cases, etc. Each ambulance building has two separate casualty dressing rooms, one for men and one for women, a ward with eight beds where sickness and accident cases can be treated at ordinary times, and where, in the event of an explosion, the victims can be promptly attended, a small emergency operating room with sterilisers for dressings and instruments and a roomy cupboard for surgical emergency appliances. At the other end of the ward there are two doctors' consulting rooms, patients' waiting room, store room, etc.

The staff of the ambulance consists of two doctors, one sister and four nurses in the shell-filling factory (where we have 7,000 workers and night shift as well as day shift) and one sister with two nurses in the cartridge-filling factory (where we have about 3,000 workers and a day shift only).

In connection with our ambulance station, we have an ambulance wagon, which is at our disposal day or night for removing patients to their homes or to hospital.

Arrangements are also made with the Local Ambulance Association for the expedition of ambulance wagons in the event of any serious explosion at the factory.

Two large local hospitals have arranged to receive our urgent cases when required in the event of explosion or otherwise. Liberal contributions are made by the factory workers to these institutions.

Any of our T.N.T. cases who have been ill enough to require hospital treatment have been sent to the . . . infirmary, where I am in touch with the Superintendent and also with the House Doctors and the Pathologist, who informs me immediately of any matter of importance concerning a worker.

CONVALESCENT HOME FOR WORKERS. The Y.W.C.A. very kindly opened a convalescent home about 6 miles from here in a bracing part of the country, and this has been kept almost entirely at our disposal and has been of inestimable value to us. The expenses of this establishment are defrayed partly by the Y.W.C.A. and partly by donations from our Workers' Hospital Fund.

HOME VISITATION OF WORKERS WHO ARE SICK. Chiefly in order to obviate the risk of girls suffering from T.N.T. poisoning lying ill at home, undiagnosed, and possibly untreated, we adopted from the beginning a system of home visitation. A post card is sent to all workers in T.N.T. parts of the factory who are reported absent for two days or more. As soon as the post card is returned asking for a visit, our health visitor calls at the house and immediately reports to me. If, as a result of this visit, it seems necessary that the doctor should call, that is done later. Girls who are in financial difficulties are assisted and infectious cases may be reported. Workers requiring subscribers' lines for admission to hospital or to convalescent home are notified, and so on. In connection with this home visiting department, we have a welfare secretary and a health visitor. The welfare secretary deals with all returned post cards. She arranges the work of the health visitor and makes reports to the doctor, keeps a card index of those visited, deals with the subscribers' lines for convalescent homes, infirmaries, etc., keeps the ' Comforts Fund ' money and the accounts connected therewith, and so on. The health visitor is not a trained nurse, but is sympathetic, tactful and conscientious, and is liked by the girls, who give her their confidence.

FINANCIAL AID TO SICK WORKERS. A fund has been in our hands for about a year and a half. The money is spontaneously voted by the workers' committee at their monthly meetings, and it is entirely subscribed by the workers themselves. Help is given from this fund to any worker who seems to be in financial distress especially through illness or accident and who is unable to provide herself with the necessary food and comfort. It is also given at times to provide holidays for necessitous cases. The money is chiefly distributed through the health visitor on the recommendation of the doctor. This system has the advantage over other systems of financial aid that is given for necessity observed by the doctors, nurses of health visitors, and does not conduce to begging.

The following is an account by a welfare officer of the arrangements which had been made at a munition works in the Midlands:

I commenced work here in 1914; for about two years I did the welfare work and nursing, but by that time the number of employees had increased so much that I had to give up the welfare work and specialise on the work I was engaged for (nursing). We have two ambulance rooms in different parts of the works but new and larger ambulance rooms with rest rooms attached are under consideration.

We are starting classes in connection with St. John Ambulance and hope to have four St. John Ambulance people—two men and two girls—in each department, in charge of an ambulance cupboard. At present all accidents are attended to by myself in the daytime and a night nurse at night. Serious cases only are sent to hospital and minor cases attended to here. Repeated dressings are done each day at the works: this is more satisfactory as it keeps us in touch with the people and we know when to expect them back at work. We also give electrical massage to those patients recommended by the doctor. Besides this I am qualified to treat simple medical cases, and we find this prevents a great loss of time by the employees. We keep a report of all accidents. All children under 16 are examined by a doctor when engaged; if they have bad teeth, a note is given them and they are sent to a dental hospital for treatment; if anything is wrong with their eyes, to the eye hospital; if anything is wrong with their throat, to the Ear and Throat hospital, and so on.

The employees pay 1d. per week and from this fund so subscribed they receive hospital notes and obtain free treatment at the hospitals. The major portion of this fund goes to the local Hospital Saturday Fund, and our employees can, when recommended by their doctor for a change of air, get a fortnight's free treatment at a convalescent home. There are two at Llandudno, one at Malvern and one at Droitwich (for Rheumatic subjects). Through the Hospital Saturday Fund our people can be supplied with artificial appliances, such as glasses and elastic stockings. The children of our workpeople obtain the same benefits, the convalescent home for the children being the Red House, Great Barr, near Birmingham. The distribution and the clerical work in connection with these notes is done entirely by the Nursing Department. The Welfare Superintendent looks the cases up and refers them all to me.

Systematic Records.

As already suggested, it is important that a full and accurate

Register should be kept of all cases of Sickness and Accident, with particulars of dressings, re-dressings and treatment.

A case book should be drawn up somewhat as follows:—

Identifi-cation number	Date	Name of injured person	Nature of injury or illness	How caused	Progress of case with dates of subsequent dressings and the occurrence of any sepsis		Date of final dressing
I	18.11.15	Mary Smith	Crushed Thumb	Fall of shell	25.11.15 30.11.15	26.11.15	3.12.15

Each case when first treated may appropriately receive a card, numbered to correspond with the entry in the case book, to be brought on the occasion of subsequent dressings.

This card must be brought to the surgery each time the patient comes for treatment.

Identification	Name	Nature of Injury	Date	Instructions
I	Mary Smith	Crushed Thumb	25.11.15.	To come tomorrow
			26.11.15.	To come on 30th.
			30.11.15.	To come on 3rd Dec.

Note: Extract from first-aid leaflet issued by the Home Office.

Treatment of Minor Injuries.
The following suggestions have the approval of H.M. Medical Inspectors of Factories in rendering first aid in factories and workshops so as to prevent subsequent septic infections or blood poisoning:

A Scratch or Slight Wound.
Do not touch it.
Do not bandage or wipe it with a handkerchief or rag of any kind.
Do not wash it.
Allow the blood to dry and so close the wound naturally, then apply a sterilised dressing and bandage.
If the bleeding does not stop, apply a sterilised dressing and sterilised wool; then bandage firmly.
If the wound is soiled with road dirt or other foul matter, swab freely with wool soaked in the iodine solution and allow the wound to dry before applying a sterilised dressing.

A Burn or Scald.
Do not touch it.
Do not wash it.
Do not apply oil or grease of any kind.
Wrap up the injured part in a large dressing of sterilised wool.

An Acid Burn.
Do not touch it, or apply oil or grease of any kind.
Flood the burn with cold water.
Sprinkle it (after flooding) with powdered bicarbonate of soda.
Apply a sterilised burn dressing of suitable size.
However slight the burn, if the area affected is extensive a doctor must be consulted.

Do not remove any dressing, but if the injured part becomes painful and begins to throb, go to a doctor at once.
Destroy all dressings which have been opened but not used; they soon become infected with microbes and then are not safe to use.
Note. Danger from minor injuries arises from blood poisoning which is caused when microbes infect a wound. The majority of wounds are at first " clean ", that is, they are not infected with microbes; such infection usually occurs later and comes from handkerchiefs or other material applied to stop bleeding or to wipe away blood, and, in the case of eye injuries, from efforts to remove fixed particles with unclean instruments. It is better to leave a wound alone than to introduce microbes by improper treatment. The congealing of blood is Nature's way of closing wounds against infection, and should not be interfered with.
Burns and scalds when the skin is not broken will heal if left alone; all that is necessary is rest and a protective covering. When blisters form they must not be pricked, except under medical advice. Rest is an important aid to healing. A short rest at first allows healing to commence and often saves a long rest later. An injured hand or finger can be rested in a sling, and an injured eye by a bandage, but an injured foot or toe can only be rested in bed.

RESULTS

The committee are satisfied of the urgent necessity and value of some such organisation as that suggested above. They have been much impressed in visiting munition works with the useful part performed by competent nurses and the large number of cases of injury and sickness which receive treatment. Thus in one munition works employing rather over 4,000 workers the ambulance department during December, 1917, dealt with 1,260 accidents (including 635 cuts, 291 bruises, and 150 eye cases), 1,703 re-dressings and 1,428 medical cases (including 415 indigestion, etc., 486 headaches and 351 colds), a total of 4,391. For January 1918, the figures were 1,186 accidents (including 670 cuts, 218 bruises and 202 eye cases), 1,956 re-dressings and 296 medical cases (including 118 indigestion, etc., 71 headaches, and 70 colds), a total of 3,438.

To sum up, it would seem appropriate to refer to the final report of the Health of Munition Workers Committee of 1918, and in particular the Section II, paragraph II, and Section III, paragraph 82, which reads:

Section II, paragraph II:

The human being is a finely adjusted physiological instrument, which must no longer be wasted, much less destroyed, by ignorant or wilful misuse. A working man's capital, is, as a rule, his health and his capacity to perform a full day's work. Once that is impaired or damaged beyond recuperation, two things happen. First, his whole industrial outlook is jeopardised and he becomes by rapid stages a liability and even a charge on the State. Secondly, if the bodily defence is undermined by stress and strain the man falls a ready prey to disease, such as tuberculosis. Therefore, as the problems to which reference is made in this report concern the future as well as the present, so also they are concerned with the new preventive medicine which has as its object the removal of the occasion of disease and physical resources of the worker in such a way and to such a degree that he can exert his full powers unhampered, and with benefit to himself and all concerned."

Section III, paragraph 82:

The national experience in modern industry is longer than that of any other people. It has shown clearly enough that false ideas of economic gain, blind to physiological law, must lead, as they led through the nineteenth century, to vast national loss and suffering. It is certain that unless industrial life is to be guided in the future—(i) by the application of physiological science to the details of its management, and (ii) by a proper and practical regard

for the health and well-being of our work-people in the form
both of humanising industry and improving the environment,
the nation cannot hope to maintain its position hereafter among
some of its foreign rivals, who already in that respect have gained
a present advantage.

No history of the many influences which have guided the
development towards better working conditions and economic
status of women in this country would be complete without
reference to the struggle for emancipation and the right to
vote which waged ferociously over the years. A quotation
from *Millicent Garrett Fawcett* by Ray Strachey, in *Great
Democrats* edited by A. Barratt Brown, gives a vivid picture
of the story:

> The turmoil of activity which centred round the suffrage
> societies went on without interruption until the very outbreak
> of the European War in August 1914, and then came to an abrupt
> standstill, or rather abruptly changed its character. Within a
> few hours of the declaration of war Mrs. Millicent Garrett Faw-
> cett had issued to her societies the call to take their share in the
> national effort. "Let us prove ourselves worthy of citizenship,
> whether our claims be recognised or not," she said, and immedi-
> ately the whole of her great organisation responded.

An intimate link with nursing and this agreement on the
part of the Suffrage Societies to bury the hatchet and to throw
themselves whole-heartedly into the war effort is brought to
mind by the pioneer work of a group of nurses and midwives
operating during the First World War in the shell factories.
Wanting to give their contribution to the health and welfare
of the munition workers, though not attracted to the more
prosaic and routine first aid and ambulance room services,
they volunteered to work as policewomen. The Women's
Police Service had come into being largely through the vision
and tenacity of Mrs. Pankhurst, Miss Damar Dawson and
Mary Allen, who attracted to their organisation an outstanding
group of well-trained women. Though largely concerned with
the enforcement of safety regulations in the filling factories

where T.N.T. poisoning took so large a toll of womanhood, this pioneer band of policewomen developed a welfare programme on broad lines and their influence could be traced to many improvements which appeared in factory life and which made conditions a little more suitable for women to endure. Work was hard and dangerous, the environment grim and unhealthy, but the appearance of the white tablecloth, or vase of flowers, cutlery and the simple necessities for a comfortable meal in the canteen, the arrangement of lockers, cloakrooms and lavatories and drinking water did much to humanise the unfamiliar surroundings where so many thousands of women and girls found themselves.

It may be difficult for younger women in industry to appreciate the battles which raged in those days on their behalf and how the green, white and purple armband of the suffragettes could have been discovered in the offices of their welfare officers had they known where to look for them. The battle colours were put into cold storage until the war was over. Then in 1917, the Representation of the People Bill, with a clause giving votes to women of thirty who were either householders or the wives of householders was passed through the House of Commons by a majority of seven to one, and early in 1918 the Bill passed the House of Lords and received Royal Assent.

In her writings at this time Mrs. Sydney Webb estimated that the average weekly wage for women in pre-First-World War days was approximately 10s. 7d. and the rapid rise in the cost of living after 1918 left them in a parlous position. Some progress had been made in 1911 when the principle of the minimum wage was granted but women generally were underpaid, sweated and exploited to an alarming degree. It was into this unhappy state of affairs that the welfare supervisor made her appearance, although in isolated industries the enlightened employer had introduced this new officer for many years. The Health of Munition Workers Committee, dealing with the Status and Duties of Welfare Supervisors, reported in these terms " any scheme of welfare supervision must be based on an adequate wage system. Without this failure is inevitable ".

It is small wonder that welfare supervisors met with constant opposition even from the workers themselves. Indeed the welfare movement generally encountered frustration, largely owing to a misconception of the aims and objects of those engaged in it. In many instances it was alleged that "welfare" was introduced to cloak the bad conditions of work; in others, that the employer used it as a " sop " to placate the underpaid workers; again that money spent on welfare schemes necessarily depressed wages and therefore was continually under suspicion.

It can, however, be said without fear of contradiction that, largely due to the high calibre of women who first entered the service, the confidence of the workers was obtained by degrees and opposition gradually lessened in intensity and in time disappeared altogether. In the early days as in more modern times it was impossible to define " welfare " and no standardised pattern could be traced through the new Service which was being developed. This lack of uniformity is perhaps its strength in that experimentation led to the wide interpretation which can be given to the early efforts to humanise industry.

Female labour selection, however, seems to be generally acknowledged as the foundation on which the service was built and the intimate confidence of the women and girls enjoyed by the supervisors gradually opened up other opportunities for service. It was the wise welfare supervisor who worked through her forewomen or chargehands in her efforts to help them.

Weird and fantastic were the underclothes worn by women during this period. Tight lacing and voluminous petticoats were in the height of fashion and mothers and grandmothers were a major problem to be dealt with by the Welfare

Supervisors because of their rigid hold on the younger generation. It is recalled how responsible women who were employed
in munition works and were called Matrons looked very
much like pincushions as they wandered round their departments—so many dangerous objects were stuck into the lapels
of their coats. Brooches, pins and hair grips were prohibited
because of the danger of explosion through friction and such
articles were confiscated if found on the girls. Particularly
difficult was it to impress upon the younger girls that "sleeper"
ear-rings, which were common wear, carried with them a
certain danger. The strong influence of mothers who upheld
the superstition that the wearing of such ear-rings from early
childhood was helpful in maintaining good eyesight, was a
serious obstacle. One resourceful "Matron" obtained a
certificate from an eminent ophthalmologist which she dis-
played in a conspicuous place in the Welfare Department,
pointing out that there was no foundation for this belief which
was so commonly held.

Welfare Supervisors in these days have amusing memories
of the varying types of womanhood who were recruited to
the munition works. Medical examinations were something
entirely new and modesty a more general virtue in those days
than at present. One Nursing Sister with a sense of humour,
throwing open the door to the doctor's room with a flourish,
when guiding in for medical examination a small under-
weight, underfed, specimen of womanhood with long wispy
locks of black hair, announced her with all the dignity at her
disposal as "Gladys Cooper". It happened, however, that
the child's name was the same as the famous actress who was
the darling of all girls at that time!

Through these influences an *esprit de corps* was developed,
inspiring loyalty to authority, to the workers themselves,
and to the job. Discipline was then foreign to the unorganised
masses, and a sense of corporate action an unknown value
under the new conditions. Through peaceful penetration,

however, headway was made. The control of environmental working conditions became the main function of the welfare supervisor. Those sections of the Factories Act concerning washing facilities, lavatories, seating accommodation and protective clothing were entrusted to her care. The running of the canteen with its attendant difficulties brought an opportunity to introduce those domestic comforts which went a long way to soften the hard and unsuitable working conditions. The clean white table cloth or vase of flowers, the orderly arrangement of the sittings, or the tidiness of the garden surrounding the dining-room all helped to cheer the drabness where so many women were forced to spend their working hours. Holidays with pay was a dream and even without pay was not the general rule. Visiting of sick absentees in hospital or at home was soon added to the duties of the welfare supervisor and this small friendly gesture no doubt went far to create a feeling of security and that someone at the factory cared. Compensation claims, always a difficult problem, sometimes came within the province of the welfare department and in the field of woman labour where shyness often prevented a claim being made, the women were protected by the vigilance of the supervisors.

Although education was a characteristic of early welfare work, very little was done on a large scale except in those factories where pioneer welfare workers had been introduced. Here a brave start had been made and although ordinary school subjects filled most of the curriculum, domestic skills such as cooking, hygiene, dressmaking, and mending were sometimes included. Club life was encouraged, and swimming, dancing, gymnastics and dramatics formed an important outlet for the use of leisure. That women should indulge in outdoor sport was, perhaps, a new idea and amusing are the pictures of the old-fashioned gym tunics or swimming suits worn by the girls at play. The modern abbreviated version of these garments is much to be recommended because of the greater appreciation now shared by women of the therapeutic value of the sun's rays on the skin.

Holiday homes and holiday camps came into being sometimes through the generosity of the firm or through voluntary effort, and the welfare supervisor recommended her girls to take full advantage of them. A wide variety of thrift and sick clubs grew spontaneously from the welfare movement. Facilities could be provided more easily on a co-operative basis and their cost controlled in consequence. The factory library, too, was an innovation. A suitable choice of books made available at little cost brought literature within easy reach of the women, the standard of which, perhaps, would not have been found elsewhere as the use of public libraries had not become so general in those days as at the present. A study of a large volume of newspaper cuttings appearing about this time discloses a repetition of the following headlines such as Welfare Work—the New Science, The Grip of the Machine, The Promotion of Industrial Peace, The New Spirit in Industry Wasting the Delicate Human Machine, The Problem of Monotony and The Human Factor. Such subjects remain equally familiar today and though much has been done, yet the problems continue to present themselves in a new guise and their solution sometimes appears as inaccessible and far away as ever in spite of the great strides which have been made. In those early days women who were truly pioneers were battling against fearful odds and as a tribute to their tenacity and indomitable courage the names of some are mentioned in this history:

The three Sisters Kerr—Miss Marie Kerr, who trained under Miss Kelly at Hudson Scott's, Carlisle, Miss C. U. Kerr, now Mrs. Cole, and Miss E. K. Kerr (the late Mrs. W. D. Wivell)— Miss Agnes Evans, S.R.N. (munition works at Gillingham, Kent and Woking), Miss Escrett, Miss Nora Wynne, Miss Frye of Woolwich Arsenal, Miss Ames (Siemens Brothers & Co., Ltd., Woolwich), and Miss Rose Pascoe, S.R.N. (Harper Bean & Co, Ltd., Dudley and Tipton, and Vickers, Sheffield), Mrs. S. B.

Aitkens, S.R.N. (Hoffman Manufacturing Co., Chelmsford), and Mrs. Barbara Lewis (Mardon, Son and Hall, Ltd., Bristol).

All these (among others unknown) helped to lay the firm foundations on which industrial welfare work has been built in some firms who were early pioneers.

It was in the midst of this " welfare " field that the factory nurse, as she was then called, found herself. In a functional management chart she was responsible to the welfare supervisor though in technical matters she was considered to be head of her department. Her position was not easy to define though the employment of a factory doctor to whom she was responsible professionally added greatly to the smooth running of her work. But full-time and part-time factory doctors were still unusual in industrial organisation. In many instances the nurse became more and more isolated from the factory itself and what was more serious still, from her profession and colleagues. She was confined to the four walls of her ambulance room, and so strictly were her movements controlled because of the fear of accidents, that meals were often taken for her to eat in isolated seclusion. Her work was considered to be first aid and first aid only. In some factories she looked after the women and not the men. It has been known for her services to be available only to the factory workers and not to the office staff. Sometimes she was allowed to care only for accidents at work and a dressing following a home or road accident was not considered her responsibility. Strange and illogical were the rules and regulations which seemed to grow up and hedge around the nurse in her ambulance room fastness. This was a phase through which she had to pass. She learned many lessons, not the least being that if her service was to develop, she must prepare herself for a richer and fuller life. Gone must be the days when knitting filled the long waiting periods between the accidents or dressing periods; gone must be the narrow interpretation which so many of the uninitiated put upon the term nursing.

The words of Lowell took on a new significance:

New times demand new measures and new men
The world advances and in time outgrows
The laws that in our fathers' days were best
And doubtless after us some purer scheme
Will be shaped out by wiser men than us
Made wise by the steady growth of truth.

During the war the Health of Munition Workers Committee published reports on a wide range of subject, and looking back in retrospect the findings and recommendations are strikingly similar to studies made in the last war. This raises the question whether many lessons learnt from 1914-1918 were forgotten and had to be re-learnt by a long and tedious struggle after 1939. Subjects on which reports and recommendations were made include: Industrial Canteens, Employment of Women, Hours of Work, Industrial Fatigue and its Causes, Sickness and Injury, Juvenile Employment, Washing Facilities and Baths, Medical Certificates, Ventilation and Lighting, Health of Munition Workers Outside the Factory.

In his memoirs Lloyd George said, "It is a strange irony that the making of weapons of destruction should afford the occasion to humanise industry. When the tumult of war is a distant echo the effects now being made will have left behind results of permanent and enduring value." On his appointment as Minister of Munitions of War, Lloyd George sent for Mr. Seebohm Rowntree, asking him to organise a welfare department within his Ministry. He suggested that welfare supervisors should be appointed in all national factories and that they should be approved by Mr. Rowntree's new department. Another name which must be woven into the survey at this juncture is that of the Rev. (now Sir) Robert Hyde, then Vicar of St. Mary's, Hoxton, later to be the founder and director of the Industrial Welfare Society. His influence on industrial welfare is widely acknowledged today. One of the results of permanent and enduring value which Lloyd George prophesied would remain " when the tumult of war is a distant echo " was the establishment in 1919 of the Welfare Workers Institute as a professional organisation and the training of these workers was developed. A quotation from *Guide to Welfare Work* by Constance Ursula Kerr, LL.D. (now Mrs. Cole), published at this time summarises the studies required of women entering this new field of social service as follows:

(a) An intimate knowledge and sympathy with women and girls. This can best be acquired by such methods as teaching in a primary school, life in a settlement, work in a women's trade union office, living at the same time in a poor neighbourhood. Without this fundamental experience no one should take up welfare work.

(b) A careful study of industrial problems which affect women's labour—such problems as the displacement of men by women, married women's work, the educational needs of " young persons " the home life of women and girls, the working of such Acts as the Insurance Acts and the Workman's Compensation Act.

(c) A knowledge, both theoretical and practical, of the health of women and girls, and how it is affected by the speed of output, the kind of commissariat provided, the question of ventilation, and heating, and questions of housing accommodation.

(d) A knowledge of the technical side of the work, indexing, filing, account keeping, domestic arrangements in rest rooms, cloak-rooms, the organisation of a factory, and the relations between general managers, foremen, and forewomen.

(e) A conception of the right relation between the life of the factory with all its agencies for good, and the life of the community, the inter-action upon the other. This involves a serious study of the social structure of the community.

In another portion of this book the author advocates the wearing of overalls because these effectually hide " V " blouses, tawdry jewellery and other unsuitable attire. Apparently the " V " blouse was a new fashion somewhat frowned upon by the welfare supervisors in those days.

It may be a far cry from the efforts of the early industrial welfare supervisors to the highly scientific studies now being carried out under the general title of a " Scientific Management " which ranges over a wide field as far apart as the psychology of conciliation and arbitration and the technique of motion study. There is, however, one common denominator which binds the two movements together—the knowledge that the human factor in industry is all important and that efficient management is the basis of all sound social development, quite apart from the more immediate question of employer-employee relationship.

It is from Seebohm Rowntree that this new science first received encouragement in this country. In 1918 he was responsible for arranging a series of week-end lecture conferences in Oxford which attracted considerable attention. At that time a new era was dawning in industry: Whitley Councils were being established and managements were beginning to evolve a new technique in their approach to the labour problems of the day. Much of the philosophy developed from these conferences was, however, inspired by earlier workers in the field and the names of Frederick Winslow Taylor (1856-1915) of U.S.A., Frank Gilbreth (1868-1924) of U.S.A., and Mary Parker Follett (1865-1933) of Boston, U.S.A., must be mentioned as pioneers. It is interesting to recall that in 1927 Mary Parker Follett spoke to industrial nurses in America, the subject of her lecture being " The Opportunities for leadership for the nurse in Industry."

In this country the name of Colonel L. Urwick, O.B.E., M.C., M.A., F.I.I.A. is remembered as an enthusiastic pioneer and a staunch advocate of these same basic principles on which the development of the " Management Movement " has been wisely built. A critical analysis of these principles has no place in this book but a quotation from the writings of Henry le Chatelier (1850-1936), a pioneer working in France, epitomises this new philosophy which was being created. Speaking of engineers he says:

" Their duty is to study the human factor of which we know

virtually nothing. Yet it is of capital importance in industry and will become continually more and more so." He did not wish to suggest that there will be no further technical progress, but merely that such progress would be achieved by methods already established. On the other hand, in dealing with the moral and social problems of industry, we have no method, we have not yet developed an established procedure, we do not know how to direct our enquiries. In this field too, we should apply scientific method. But the problem is a complex one. . . . In short the study of the many different aspects of the human factor in industry demands special methods."

He then went on to analyse the place of the human factor in production, that is to say scientific management, and in commerce, that is to say economic science, and added:

" These two disciplines of scientific management and economics only deal with the human factor from the material point of view of production and exchange. But it must also be studied from the angle of human needs. It is not enough to secure a maximum output, we must also pay attention to the principles of justice. And that is the province of a third discipline, morals."

Having outlined some of the difficulties of applying scientific method of moral problems, he concluded:

" Let us hope, without cherishing illusions, that if the nineteenth century remains famous in human history for progress in experimental science and for the creation of large-scale industry, the twentieth century in its turn will be noted for its understanding of social problems and for its love of justice. At least let us dedicate ourselves to this purpose."

5

Industry and the Home Nursing Service

ALTHOUGH Philippa Flowerday, the first industrial nurse, was both district nurse and factory nurse, it is not always remembered how close was the connection between district nursing and industry in the early days. For example, an unusual and very personal service was supplied to the industrial worker through the imagination of the Belper Humane Society established in 1824. This Society later came to be closely associated with the Belper Nursing Association and as recently as 1927 issued a joint report.

The rules of the Society were:

1. That this Society shall have for its object the supply of clean linen to the sick poor of the Township of Belper free of expense.

2. That the Committee shall appoint a female to deliver the linen to the sick, to receive it from them, disinfect the same, and forward it without delay to Messrs. Strutt, who have kindly engaged that it shall be washed at their Bleach Yard at the smallest possible expense.

3. That a Certificate from a Medical Attendant or District Nursing Association Nurse, addressed to the female having care of the linen, shall in all cases be sufficient to entitle the Sick to the benefit of the Society. The Certificate to be renewed at the end of four weeks, if the supply of linen is to be continued.

4. That the Medical men of the Town, in fever or other extreme cases, be authorised to order the room or rooms of any patient to be cleansed by a charwoman, who shall be paid by the Society an adequate fee, and also in urgent need order a nurse for a period not exceeding eight days, by a note to the Hon. Secretary.

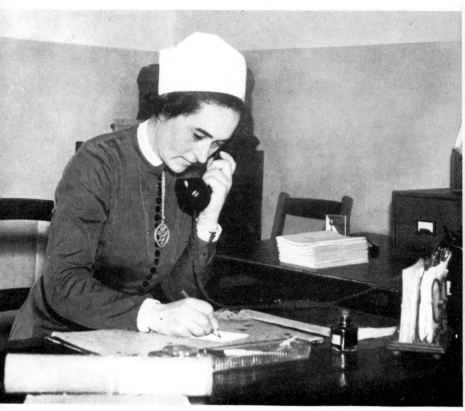

A QUEEN'S SUPERINTENDENT KEEPS THE LINK BETWEEN
THE FACTORY AND THE HOME

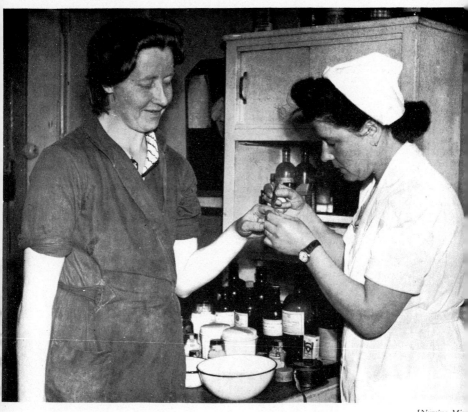

[*Nursing Mir*

CONCENTRATION

The firm of Strutt, whose mills are on the banks of the Derwent, later became the English Sewing Cotton Company and the wide sympathetic interest of Lord and Lady Belper is reflected in the philanthropic and cultural improvements the family has made in this beautiful Derbyshire valley.

There have also been many isolated experiments for the provision of nurses to work with the miners at the pit head and to follow them into their own homes during illness. Such services were generally supported from a levy stopped out of wages. Sometimes this was supplemented by money from the mine owners and much later grants from the Miners' Welfare Fund brought district nursing to many mining villages. An interesting example of such a comprehensive health scheme comes from Yorkshire and these early beginnings were later amalgamated into the Edlington and Warmsworth Nursing Association. The benefits to the miners who subscribed 6d. a week included:

(a) medical and home nursing for the whole family.
(b) pit head baths.
(c) large donations to local hospitals.
(d) grants to Rheumatic Clinic at Buxton.
(e) the provision of artificial limbs.
(f) transport to hospital.
(g) social recreation for the family.
(h) convalescent home service.

Although little is known of the work of Philippa Flowerday, yet it is on record that she spent the morning in the factory and the afternoon in the home, this no doubt being the ideal interpretation of any industrial nursing service. In modern times, however, when specialisation is necessary, separate services must be maintained. But it is only through close co-operation between the two nursing groups that a complete service can be given to the community. This co-operation has now developed and extended to other public health nurses working in the home such as the health visitors, tuberculosis visitors, school nurse, midwives and nursery matrons. Each group as a member of the health team brings its own particular experience to bear on the service to be given in the home. The industrial nurse is now accepted as a member of the public health team and the service she can give is a valuable link in forging the specialist public health services into a whole.

To encourage this co-operation between the industrial and district nurse the Central Bureau for Insurance Nursing was established in 1929. The Central Bureau was formed as a professional organisation responsible for administering a home nursing service offered, free of charge, to their policy holders by the Mutual Property Insurance Company Ltd. now the Crusader Insurance Company Limited, and the Metropolitan Life Insurance Company of New York. Among other things the Bureau encouraged the reference of patients by the industrial nurse employed in firms holding a group insurance policy with either of these Companies to the appropriate District Nursing Associations throughout the country.

The main objects of the Central Bureau were:

1. The home nursing and health education of policy-holders of the participating companies.
2. The establishment of medical and nursing services within industrial and commercial concerns.
3. To foster closer co-operation between industry and the public health nursing services.

In order to ensure the routine " follow-up " of all absence due to sickness, " automatic notification " to the district nurse was encouraged and in order to assist the factory medical departments in placing calls in London and elsewhere, call offices were established for receiving nursing calls and relaying them to the various Nursing Associations.

A " standing order " endorsed by the British Medical Association regularised this procedure. It stated:

It is permissible for a call to be given to a nurse by any responsible person, but under no circumstances shall more than two visits be made by her unless a doctor is in attendance. If a call is sent to a nurse by anyone other than a doctor and on her visit she advises a doctor should be called, but on her second visit finds her advice has not been taken, she shall discontinue attending the case.

Since the inception of this service up to July 5, 1948, when home nursing became the responsibility of the State through the facilities of the National Health Service, approximately 786,000 home nursing visits were made to industrial workers or their families by the many thousands of Queen's, Ranyard and other District Nurses in the field. The value of this work, which brought comfort and advice to so many homes, cannot be measured, but the satisfaction to the nurse, the response of her patients and their families and the service rendered to the employers are proof enough that a useful service was available. An object lesson in the value of close co-operation between the factory and the home in cases of sickness and disablement was demonstrated.

Speaking to a group of public health nurses in America in 1922, Dr. Louis I. Dublin, Ph.D., Statistician, Metropolitan Life Insurance Company of New York said: " The newer health activities will depend very largely on the nursing profession for personnel. To be most effective and to realise her highest opportunities the nurse must see the relation of her work to the larger purposes of the community. She must be a student of sickness; she must take a professional attitude to her work, and not be content with routine procedures alone. She must see the new implications in her many-sided work. It is for this reason that records are developed and it is through their proper use that these developments may be achieved". It was with this object in view that the Central Bureau developed a record system for use among District Nursing Associations which was designed by experts in consultation with the nurses, in order to meet their particular needs. Furthermore, advice and assistance was available through the Bureau for factories who were contemplating the installation of health records in their Medical Departments. A careful analysis was made of all records of insured patients nursed in their own homes, which were sent to the Bureau for payment; the findings raised many professional points for discussion and subsequent action. For instance, it was found that the sepsis rate remained fairly constant over the years. Approximately 10 per cent of all cases referred to the district nurses through the Bureau were for " septic " conditions. This presented a problem for serious study and a critical enquiry revealed that in some instances professional technique may have been in error. Other factors concerned in the problem were also discovered and attention directed to them. The first step, however, was to establish the facts and later to take steps to consider them in relation to the matter under review.

We need only to recall the numerous reforms instituted by Florence Nightingale in order to appreciate her unusual ability to reason from the individual cases of sickness she met in the hospital or the home to the general principles underlying sickness and disability. Her interest in this matter was aroused from the first statistical reports published by the Government in this country, following the investigations of Dr. Farr, who spoke of his work as " his little sums about human lives ". From her study of these reports Miss Nightingale learned that the death rate in the first year of life was 227 per thousand in the Counties of Staffordshire, Shropshire and in Leeds, where the investigations were made. This inspired her to question the causes underlying the social conditions of her day. Later in her career she sought the reason for the many deaths in the military hospitals in the Crimea and among the population of India. "What sanitary failure was responsible for hospital infections?" she asked. Much of the brilliance of Miss Nightingale's work was due to her outstanding ability to interpret records. This, no doubt, was due to her lifelong habit of probing collected official reports and records of sickness and of installing good systems where they did not exist. Although she was never in India, yet from reports and statistics kept by the Government there, she was able to point to defects in sanitary arrangements which, when rectified, brought far-reaching improvements in the health of that country. Florence Nightingale appreciated and taught that a nurse was not fulfilling her whole duty to her patients if she failed to reflect upon the causes and prevention of sicknesss and if she did not keep good records or failed to study them earnestly.

Without the careful and intensive work steadily carried out by industrial nurses through World War II much of the enquiry then made into the causes of absence due to sickness in industry would not have been collected and such figures are invaluable. The industrial nurse doing work of this nature may feel that it could be undertaken satisfactorily by a suitably trained clerk, but she should remember that the information on the health card is of a confidential nature.

The various forms of medical or health records to be kept by the Health Departments in Industry were much debated during the early days of the war and in 1944 the Medical Research Council published a preliminary report by a Sub-Committeee of the Industrial Health Research Board No. 85. This report gives the main objects for the keeping of health records as follows:

1. To obtain knowledge of the health of the individual worker in order to see if he or she is fit for the work; to assist allocation or transfer to the work for which he or she is best fitted; and to determine, if possible, whether work undertaken is having any ill effects on health.
2. To collect information about the health of groups of workers within each organisation, in order to find out whether particular conditions of methods of work have any ill effects on health.
3. To collect information about the health of groups of workers throughout the country, engaged on similiar or related work.
4. To provide information on the collective health of all industrial workers.
5. To assess the value of measures applied to reduce the incidence of sickness.

6. To provide essential data for research into problems of industrial health.

The Report also discusses the best methods for collecting the necessary data for compiling the statistics. A suitable card, chiefly designed to record in a simple way absences due to sickness and other causes, was evolved and industrial nurses entered wholeheartedly into the experiment. Their comments, valuable because they were based on actual practical use in daily routine, were of considerable assistance to the research authorities who were compiling statistics on current topics and at the same time working out simple methods for collecting them. In this respect the research carried out by the Industrial Safety Division of the Royal Society for the Prevention of Accidents has been of great assistance in that a classification, based on that used by the Factory Department of the Ministry of Labour and National Service, is now generally accepted and is a simple method by which the industrial nurse can make her analysis of lost time due to accidents and disease.

In January 1948 a first organised move was made in Manchester to consider ways and means for bringing about better co-operation between the district nurses and industrial nurses in that city. The subject was on the agenda of the Industrial Nurses Group of the Public Health Section within the Manchester Branch of the Royal College of Nursing. The meeting, representative of industrial nurses and Queen's nurses, welcomed the opportunity to meet and discuss so important a matter. It was recalled that in many of the early industrial nursing experiments the industrial nurse had followed her patients into their homes to give home nursing care and in this way a complete service was given. In later days the more specialised services which had developed had tended to wind along parallel roads lined with high hedges, and overlapping and lack of co-operation prevented the best being available for those in need. It was agreed that the modern approach to all such problems was through enlightened co-operation and good team work, for only in that way could there be full efficiency in any field of human endeavour.

The meeting agreed to set up a " Working Party " of Queen's nurses and industrial nurses in the Manchester area, to consider in detail how such co-operation could be developed. A survey of the local firms employing industrial nurses was made and information of the available facilities for home nursing supplied to them. In the field of home nursing the facts relating to industrial nursing were brought to the district nurse's notice and slowly but surely the spirit of co-operation is being diffused around the groups which can but have a helpful effect on the welfare of the patient and his nursing care during sickness or disability at home.

At this meeting the following resolution was passed and submitted to the Public Health Section of the Royal College of Nursing:

> Realising that the Industrial Health Service is not at present an integral part of the National Health Service, and that only by close co-operation within the health team can the best service for industry be produced, and realising that many anomalies exist in public health nursing practice, this meeting of the Industrial Nurses Group of the Public Health Section within the Manchester Branch of the Royal College of Nursing, at which many Queen's Nurses are visitors, asks the Public Health Section to encourage free discussion among the Sections on how best to co-operate within the Service and to draw up recommendations for the members' guidance.

Considerable interest on this important point was aroused in the country and from this beginning new approaches to the problem are being developed with satisfactory results.

6

Dark Days Between the Wars

THE brave beginning made by Industrial Nursing in the First World War received a serious set-back when peace came. In many cases employers had looked upon the new service as an expensive luxury and, when the axe of economy made retrenchment necessary, this service, like others which had hitherto rested on firm foundations, had to be curtailed, if not entirely abolished. These were dark, black days. Little is recorded on this period but it is known that the trained nurse in many cases gave place to other ancillary grades.

Some industrial nursing experiments had, however, become firmly established and the following firms may be mentioned as pioneers in the field:

Cadbury Bros., Bournville; C. Kunzle Ltd., Birmingham; Rowntree & Co. Ltd., York; W. D. & H. O. Wills Ltd., Bristol; The Co-operative Wholesale Society Ltd.; Jas. Templeton & Son Ltd., Glasgow; J. Lyons & Co. Ltd., Cadby Hall; British Xylonite Co. Ltd., London; Geo. Garnett & Sons Ltd., Bradford; J. S. Fry & Sons Ltd., Bristol; Reckitt & Sons, Hull; Wm. Beardmore & Co. Ltd., Glasgow; David Brown & Sons Ltd., Huddersfield; Morgan Crucible Co. Ltd., Battersea; Kodak Ltd., Wealdstone; Stanton Ironworks Co. Ltd., Nottingham; Mardon, Son & Hall Ltd., Bristol; Hoffman Manufacturing Co. Ltd., Chelmsford; Debenham and Freebody, Ltd.

There were, however, some new ventures during this period and in 1925 the Mutual Property Insurance Company Limited, now the Crusader Insurance Company Limited, appointed a part-time doctor and a State-registered nurse to look after the health of their staff at their London headquarters. From the commencement of this service a complete physical examination was offered to all employees, such an interpretation of " prevention is better than cure " being somewhat unusual at that time. It is believed this company was the first commercial firm to establish a comprehensive health service for its staff. The company also developed a unique piece of industrial nursing through the provision of home nursing for their industrial and group policy-holders, the actual service being given through the District Nursing Association. This has been described in Chapter 5.

In another direction also a new beginning was made in the establishment of a Ships' Nursing Service. Prior to 1927 trained nurses had been employed by some shipping companies in the capacity of a stewardess or conductress. This was usually their policy if a large emigrant population was carried, particularly on the long voyages to Australia and New Zealand. In the case of the Cunard Steamship Company Ltd. some nurses were first employed about this time as stewardesses on the cruising ships and in between these duties they sailed in charge of the ship's hospital and were known as " matrons ". In January 1927, however, these women were given the status of Nursing Sisters and a rapid development in the nursing service took place so that before the year was out each Cunard liner carried a State-registered nurse. In this history of nursing development it is interesting to mention, wherever possible, the names of pioneers in their special fields, and in this respect the name of Miss Grace Medlock of the Cunard Steamship Co. Ltd. can be recorded. She sailed up to the time the Sisters were taken off the ships, early in the Second World War.

In the pioneer days the Medical Department of the Anchor Line was directed under the supervision of the Medical Superintendent of the Cunard Steamship Company Ltd., and Nursing Sisters served on the S.S. *California* and the S.S. *Caledonia*. Other companies carrying Nursing Sisters are

Canadian Pacific Steamships Ltd., Blue Star Line, Booth Steamship Co. (London) Ltd., Orient Line, and New Zealand Shipping Co. Ltd. With reference to the last-mentioned company, Nursing Sisters were carried on the Canadian-New Zealand run as early as 1924. It is now an accepted practice that generally speaking Nursing Sisters are established as members of the ship's company.

An average-sized liner, carrying a complement of 2,000 passengers and crew, presents an interesting field for public health nursing and attracts a woman of wide experience, for a knowledge of the world is essential for meeting the many problems which present themselves on a ship in mid-ocean. Her duties are many and varied, for the ship's crew, so often out of sight in the engine room and below deck, are comparable in many ways to the industrial workers in a factory and are her concern in the same way that the passengers come under her care. Her daily clinic routine differs in no way from the out-patients' department of a hospital or a surgery at a factory. The problems of human nature are the same on land as on sea and it is a tribute to the Shipping Companies that a high standard of service is now available through Nursing Sisters on nearly all vessels whether on the regular routes or on luxury cruises.

7

Industrial Nursing Organisation

In the year 1881, Annie Cass, the daughter of Sir John Cass of Bradford, was married to Weetman Pearson, the son of George Pearson, of the firm of S. Pearson and Son, operating round Huddersfield in the contracting and building trade. It had early been discovered that young Weetman Pearson was no ordinary lad and his father sent him on an extensive tour so that he might see the world before settling down in the family business. On his return from his travels a party was arranged for him to show the treasures which he had brought back from Palestine. Among them was a Bible bound in olive wood which he offered to Annie Cass, one of the guests, announcing that the gift was intended for the woman he would make his wife. She was then seventeen and refused the gift, tossing her head and calling him a cheeky boy, but a year later he declared his intention once more and was readily accepted. A perfect partnership was thus begun, and after Lord Cowdray's death (for the passage of years had made many changes in the Pearson fortunes) two days before he was to have received the Freedom of Aberdeen, his intended reply to the honour was printed in the *Aberdeen Press* of May 3rd, 1927. It contained these words: " Nothing comes into the same category with the great crowning influence which a man possesses in that perfect partner, a well mated wife. To have by you one who shares with head and heart, the successes and the failures, who gives due encouragement but has the courage to administer the home truths, unpalatable but necessary sometimes, who is never afraid of responsibility, prepared to start life afresh should need arise, such a partner is beyond praise or price. She is simply one's needed life blood and I make no apology, my Lord Provost, for this due tribute to mine." Lady Cowdray for her part, in the course of her reply, for she went alone to Aberdeen, said: "From our joint start in life it seems to me that we two settled, almost without knowing it, two of the burning questions of the day which are still agitating many minds. The first is "Is woman's place necessarily limited to the home?" The second, "Should married women work?" I shall eternally be thankful that life gave me a partner who answered both these questions in my own spirit. To that freedom, my Lord Provost, I owe today's Freedom, if in any sense at all I have any claim to deserve it at your hands."

We must go back to the early days of the firm when contract after contract poured into the rapidly expanding organisation. An office was opened at Delahay Street in London which Mrs. Pearson furnished down to the smallest detail and she and her husband spent Saturday afternoons together tidying up after the staff had gone home. Success followed their efforts and vast civil engineering contracts were undertaken—drainage and sewage works, reservoirs, harbour and dock construction, railways, canals and tunnels, largely for British and foreign governments. Extensive city development schemes also, at home and abroad, were undertaken with great success.

No work was too difficult for Weetman Pearson, the intrepid young civil engineer who was now head of the firm. One of his firmest principles was that he would never ask his men to go where he would not venture himself and, when exceptional engineering difficulties were met in the construction of the tunnel under the Hudson River in New York, he himself fell victim to the dreaded compressed-air or caisson disease, known to the workers as the "bends" or the "blind staggers ". This disease occurs when the return to normal air pressure, after working in compressed air, is made too quickly. If the external air pressure is allowed to drop too suddenly the air which has been taken into the body under pressure is absorbed into the tissues, and this causes damage, especially to the tissues of the brain and the spinal cord. There is violent pain in the limbs followed by paralysis and cerebral disturbances. This disease had appeared as a result of the modern use of compressed air and had been described during the building of the Forth Bridge.

In December 1890, Mr. Pearson insisted on going into the region of high air pressure under the Hudson River and became paralysed from the waist down within forty-five minutes of coming to the surface. The Pearson firm had been studying the aetiology and treatment of this condition and had established, above ground and near the entrance to the shaft, medical treatment centres containing airlocks. These centres were fitted with beds and provided with nursing comforts, and were lighted with electricity. They were staffed by a doctor and nurses, and Mrs. Pearson had carefully supervised development of this new industrial health service. Men seized with the " bends " were carried to the medical airlock and, the airtight door having been closed, the pressure was again raised to somewhere near that at which the men had been working and was then very gradually reduced to the normal. Patients were taken into these airlocks paralysed and acutely ill but, after about an hour in the pressure chambers most of them walked away in a normal state of health. The death rate dropped from this condition from 25 per cent to $1\frac{1}{2}$ per cent. It was into such an airlock that Mr. Pearson was taken and, although his condition was serious, with the careful nursing by his wife and her nurses, he recovered, though he was forbidden by his doctors to expose himself to high pressure again.

Since the labour force used by the firm was largely Irish and was migratory in habits, encampments were built to accommodate large numbers of men and their wives near to the site of each constructional work. Mrs. Pearson personally supervised the " welfare " arrangements at these encampments and a doctor and nurse were appointed to look after the health of each community. Temporary hutments were built, sanitary services were improved and clean water was brought to the site. Feeding arrangements, hot drinks and the provision of blankets were not forgotten and it is on record that the men expressed the opinion that, owing to Mrs. Pearson's forethought and practical organising ability, the comfort of the workers had been greatly improved and much ill health had been prevented.

Recognising the great need existing for helping the large number of navvies engaged on the vast constructional works going on all over the country, Mrs. Elizabeth Garnett had founded the Navvies' Mission Society in 1877. Mr. and Mrs. Pearson generously supported this enterprise, which provided navvies' schools, libraries and religious activities. The Aged Navvies' Pension Fund was founded in the Pearson home and continued for 25 years until the state pension fund made this unnecessary. Mrs. Pearson was both president and treasurer of the Fund.

Many of the civil engineering enterprises completed by the firm were in tropical countries—Vera Cruz, Egypt, Mexico, Chile and the Sudan—where tropical diseases took a heavy toll of the labour force. Water was often contaminated and mosquitoes and sandflies carried hidden diseases. Mr. Pearson encouraged research into the cause of yellow fever and malaria and in many ways pioneered in the early conquest of these diseases. It was proved that much of the malarial infection could be traced to mosquito bites suffered by men taking their siestas unprotected in daylight. A rule was therefore made enforcing, at all times, the use of those methods of protection which had formerly been adopted to prevent the men being bitten at night. Mr. Pearson was always careful of the health and comfort of his men, for he recognised that good housing, pure water and clean food, with medical aid at hand, were an absolute necessity if he was not to be beaten by disease among his workers. He was not unmindful of the recent experiences of de Lesseps and his engineers who were ruined in their efforts to build a canal across the Isthmus of Panama, so malaria ridden was the country in which they had to work.

Pearson always looked upon the building of the Tehuantepec Railway in Mexico as the finest and most difficult achievement of the firm. Since 1550, when the Portuguese navigator, Antonio Gavao, published a book to show that a canal could be cut to link the Atlantic and Pacific Oceans, there had been discussion as to the best route across the isthmus. The Spanish Government had a plan, the Americans conceived others, but all to no avail. Pearson firmly believed the best plan practicable was for the complete reconstruction of the existing inadequate and unserviceable railway: in addition deep water ports on the Atlantic and Pacific coasts would have to be constructed. Despite overwhelming difficulties he persevered and, with the close co-operation of President Diaz of Mexico, at last completed the contract. The Tehuantepec railway across the isthmus was opened on January 25th, 1907, the whole of Mexico being in gala mood for the occasion.

It was in 1910 that Mr. Pearson was raised to the peerage in the title of Baron Cowdray of Midhurst. One of his earliest benefactions thereafter was the gift of the Cowdray Hospital to Mexico City. In connection with this hospital a district nursing service was set up. Lady Cowdray took the deepest interest in this work, and her attention to detail, her power of organisation, and her deep understanding of the needs of a hospital and its patients, were all brought to bear on planning a first class hospital for Mexico City. Later Lord Cowdray turned his attention to prospecting for oil in Mexico and a vast fortune was made from this source.

The largest operation carried out by the firm during the 1914 war was the building of the great munition town of Gretna which was established in order to make good, in the least possible time, the shortage of high explosives that had existed in the early days of the war.

Lady Cowdray had unceasingly interested herself in nursing matters and round her homes in Aberdeenshire and Sussex she had long supported district nurses—at one time there were no fewer than seven " Queen's Nurses " working at her expense. The first World War brought nursing into prominence, largely because of the great work which was done so quietly on many battlefronts, and many thinking men and women realised that something must be done to improve the conditions to which the nurses would return when the war was over and the enthusiasm had died away. Some Nurses would return wounded and disabled. There was no organisation to receive them or to lighten the burden of disablement and prolonged illness resulting from the war. Furthermore there was no roll on which the trained nurse could place her name and statistics about the country's nursing force were lacking. To the older members of the nursing profession much of this story will be familiar but the younger generation, who are receiving the benefit of the forethought and wisdom of the pioneers, may not quite realise all that has been done for them. It is to that great friend of nurses, the late Sir Arthur Stanley, that our thoughts must first turn. As Chairman of the British Red Cross Society, he could see the difficulties which nurses would face. Together with the Matron-in-Chief of the Society, Dame Sarah Swift, he consulted with Sir Cooper Perry, then Medical Superintendent of Guy's Hospital, and arranged a meeting to which leaders of the profession were called. The object of the meeting was to form an organisation " whose policy should be to unite all trained nurses in an endeavour to provide a uniform standard of training which should be a basis of membership of a College; to improve the quality of the nursing service and the conditions under which nurses work; to assist in procuring State registration of nurses and to further in every possible way the advancement of the profession through legislation, post-graduate study, theoretical and practical scholarships and specialised training". St. Thomas's Hospital was the scene of the meeting.

It was soon discovered that money in large amount would be needed to carry out the plans which were evolving. There was in existence at the time a British Women's Hospital Committee which had raised large funds to build the Star & Garter Home at Richmond for totally disabled men. To someone came the happy thought that perhaps this Committee would continue their work and endow a College of Nursing and also consider the founding of a benevolent fund which was so urgently needed to help nurses coming home from the war. Dame May Whitty was the Chairman of the Appeal. Miss Lilian Braithwaite acted as Hon. Secretary and Viscountess Cowdray was Hon. Treasurer. The large sum of £148,915 was soon collected. Lady Cowdray's personal gifts through the fund reflected her practical approach to any problem, for she endowed scholarships and two Cowdray pensions for disabled nurses; but that was not the end. Miss Rachel Cox-Davies, Matron of the Royal Free Hospital, was a woman to whom Lady Cowdray could always turn for advice on the needs of nurses and she inspired other projects. A social club to provide a centre for intercourse, which should furnish some of those creature comforts associated with the word " home ", was Lady Cowdray's happy inspiration and No. 20 Cavendish Square, once the home of Mr. and Mrs. Herbert Asquith was bought and presented to the College of Nursing. Later, the rebuilding of adjoining sites which had been bought by the College was undertaken as a result of further gifts of Lord and Lady Cowdray. Nurses who frequent the handsome head-quarters in Henrietta Place, W.1, have cause to be ever grateful to their great benefactor who not only provided the large sums of money which were needed, but also personally supervised the delightful decorations of the buildings.

The College of Nursing in 1923 established a Public Health Section and nurses who were College members engaged in one or other of the public health and preventive nursing services were eligible for membership. In an annual report published by the Section in 1929 an interesting note appears—probably the first reference to industrial nurses as an organised body. It reads: " Efforts are being made to ascertain the conditions under which nurses employed in factories or business houses are working and members are asked to send in any useful information they can obtain." The response could not have been too encouraging because in the following year the annual report gave another reminder, saying " very little information is reaching us with regard to industrial nurses. It seems to be work with great possibilities and absorbing interest but we have little knowledge. We should be so grateful if nurses doing this work would collect as much information as they can and send it on to us."

In April 1928 the first National Conference on Industrial Nursing was called by the Industrial Welfare Society and took place at the Hotel Metropole, London. The arrangements were made by Mrs. C. U. Cole of the Women's and Girls' Department of the Society and it is largely due to her enthusiasm and appreciation of the wide scope and function of the industrial nurse that the success of the Conference was assured. Over 100 delegates attended. Sir Edward M. Iliffe, M.P., and Lady Dawson of Penn were guests of the Conference and in the evening the delegates went to the Garrick Theatre, where "The Lady with the Lamp ", by Reginald Berkeley, was being played.

The programme included papers on the following subjects:

"Industrial Nursing—its Scope and Possibilities ", by Mrs. C. U. Cole, L.L.A. (Hons.)

" My Work as a Factory Nurse ", by Miss M. J. S. Boswell, S.R.N., Kodak Ltd., Wealdstone.

" Nursing in Relation to Industrial Welfare ", by Dr. Margaret L. Dobbie-Bateman, Medical Officer, Harrods Ltd.

" Co-operation between the Welfare Superintendent and the Nurse ", by Miss E. K. Kerr, Carreras Ltd.

" Nursing in Relation to Industrial Welfare ", by Dr. Leonard Lockhart, Medical Officer, Boots Pure Drug Co.

A quotation from this latter paper summarises the position of the nurse in industry at the time and may be taken as a point of view held generally by the medical and nursing professions at that date:

After more than a decade of very active health and welfare development, we find that industry is still unable to attract to its immediate service a sufficient supply of the nation's best nurses. Not only have we difficulty in persuading nurses to take up this work, but we have difficulty in extending its scope so as to make it a vital and energising spark in the health services of the country.

As far as the nurses themselves are concerned, we must remember that their training and outlook centres, in the main, on the curative branch of medicine. Small wonder, then, that the desire to carry on in the curative branch of their profession becomes to so many an absorbing passion; so that when promotion threatens to engulf them in the official side of hospital administration there are always those who will set it aside in order to take up some duty, however onerous or poorly paid, where they can be sure that the sick bed will never become subordinate in their minds to the office. These are the women whom we try to tempt into the ranks of preventive medicine, nor shall we ever succeed unless and until we are in a position to offer them the only inducement which will bring them to consider the question.

Preventive medicine can become dull, but it can quite easily take on another aspect altogether, and there is no doubt that we have allowed nurses to believe for too long that of all uninteresting work the industrial branch of preventive medicine is quite the most dull. The prevention of ill-health and disability, the early treatment of manifest disease and the prevention of as much as possible of what remains is without exception our most pressing and urgent duty. We have allowed preventive medicine for so

long to be graded low in the scale of things that matter. I believe
that many a nurse on taking service in industry has felt that she
has to some extent burnt her professional boats or at least made
them distinctly unseaworthy.

On the other hand we find that industry has not set out to make
its appointments as attractive as it should; and this is very largely
because its eyes are as yet fully opened neither to the value and
scope of preventive medicine, nor to the aspirations and capabilities of the nurses which it finds itself called upon to employ.

. . . We need to see more virility and more energy put into this
matter of industrial nursing. We need to see an adequate supply
of nurses and we need to see them used to the best advantage.
It is necessary for us to arouse interest among employers, to enlist
the support and co-operation of the nurses' training schools and
to supply that additional training in the factory which will enable
the good sick nurse to become the efficient instrument of
economic well-being which we all know she can be.

The Rev. (now Sir) R. R. Hyde, then Director of the
Industrial Welfare Society, took the chair at the Conference
and read a message to the Assembly from the Duke of York,
later King George VI. In his introductory remarks he said:

" The Conference which now begins is but another link in the
chain of progress of a comparatively modern movement. All
progress is brought about by the secession of a part of a body in
order to develop in a separate field of existence. Here new technique is acquired; practitioners are trained; fresh codes and
standards of practice are set up and those engaged in this new
enterprise exchange views upon matters of common interest.
For the first time in history industrial nursing is recognising
itself in these ways in a conference representative of practically
every industry in the country."

During 1928 joint discussions on the place of the trained nurse
in industry continued between the Public Health Section of the
College of Nursing, the Industrial Welfare Society and the
Institute of Industrial Welfare Workers, and an early report
states that the subjects under consideration were:

(a) The status of the trained nurse in industry.
(b) Training required in addition to hospital experience.
(c) Remuneration.

(*d*) Present scope of work—its possible extension on the lines of preventive medicine.

(*e*) Advisability of combining industrial welfare work with industrial nursing in smaller factories and industries.

The same report states that the average salary offered to a trained nurse in industry was at that time £3 a week.

On October 3, 1932, at 2 p.m., a meeting was called at the College of Nursing, Henrietta Street (now Henrietta Place), W.1, the notice convening the meeting stating simply, "To consider the position of nurses in industry". The meeting agreed to set up a committee of nurses, the following being the first members:

Miss Olive Baggallay, S.R.N., Chairman, Public Health Section.
Miss Boswell, S.R.N. (the first Chairman appointed), Sister-in-Charge, Kodak Ltd., Wealdstone.
Miss Cardozo, S.R.N., Superintendent Health Visitor, Poplar.
Miss Carol Mann, S.R.N., Welfare Supervisor, Wolsey Ltd., Leicester.
Miss K. Roe, S.R.N., Health Visitor, Royal Borough of Kensington.
Miss B. Shenton, S.R.N., Sister-in-Charge, Staff Welfare Dept., Mutual Property Insurance Co. Ltd.
Miss E. Hopkins, S.R.N.
Miss A. Evans, S.R.N., Superintendent, Willesden District Nursing Association.
Miss I. H. Charley, S.R.N., Hon. Secretary, Public Health Section ; Nursing Superintendent, Mutual Property Insurance Company Ltd.
Miss F. E. Udell, S.R.N., Secretary to the Public Health Section.
Mrs. C. U. Cole, L.L.A., Industrial Welfare Society.

The first matter to be considered was a suitable training for industrial nurses and it was reported that in the opinion of the Committee an ideal preparation for this new branch of public health nursing would be the six months Health Visitors Course suitably adapted to meet the requirements of industry. It was stressed that as there was so much in common between the district nursing service and nursing in industry a proportion of the time—not less than one month—should be spent with a district nurse.

The Secretary was asked to confer with the Home Office, the Industrial Welfare Society, and the Institute of Labour Management (formerly the Institute of Industrial Welfare Workers) on the plans the College were making. At the second meeting the interest and sympathy of these bodies was reported, particularly the Home Office, which had suggested that the College should arrange an intensive course of study for nurses already engaged in factories.

It was recommended that the scale of salaries suggested by the College for health visitors should be applied to industrial nurses and that protest should be made to employers where the salary offered was less than £200 a year. Certain other fundamental principles were elaborated: the nurse should be recognised as a professional woman directly responsible to the Board of Directors; she should be paid a salary and not a wage; she should not be required to pay unemployment insurance; she should be allowed to remain in the Federated Super-annuation Scheme for Nurses and Hospital Officers (Contributory), and, if she were already a member, her employer should pay his appropriate share of contributions.

In order to discover facts about the employment of industrial nurses in the country a questionnaire was sent out to 125 nurses known to be working in this field and 38 were returned. It is amusing to note that in response to this enquiry a reply came from nurses working in the Coventry area expressing the opinion that £250 a year, the College scale, was too high a salary to be asked and that Industry would not pay it. Perhaps no such resolution either before or since, in any field of human endeavour, has ever been passed.

In 1932 the writer was asked to read a paper at a Conference of the Royal Institute of Public Health in Belfast, the title being " A Contribution by the Insurance World to Industrial Health ". The late Sir Thomas Oliver, M.A., M.D., D.Sc.,

LL.D., D.L.O., F.R.C.P., Professor of Principles and Practice of Medicine, University of Durham and College of Medicine, Newcastle upon Tyne, well known for his research into the dangers of lead and phosphorus, was in the chair, but so little interest was taken in this subject at that time that, when the writer came to speak, only the Chairman and two other industrial medical officers were present, the rest of the audience having drifted away to lunch. But those remaining, Mr. T. E. A. Stowell, M.D., F.R.C.S., and Dr. H. B. Trumper, M.A., M.B., B.Chir.(Cantab.), then both of Imperial Chemical Industries, were interested in what she had to say and tribute is here given to the great encouragement they gave her in those early days. It is also a pleasure to mention Dr. Leonard Lockhart who, by his unfailing sympathy and enthusiasm, did much to encourage industrial nurses in the pioneering days.

Industrial nurses by this time were emerging from their seclusion, many of them having been tucked away for years in a surgery, perhaps only tolerated because the Factories Act required a " responsible person trained in first aid " to be available in case of accidents. They were now asking for special preparations for their work and were feeling the need for professional contact with their nursing colleagues. Popular weekend courses were arranged by the College of Nursing in London, Nottingham, Manchester, Liverpool and Leeds, and medical officers and industrialists gave generously of their time to provide useful and interesting programmes.

The first effort towards professional organisation was to make a survey of the country and in diverse ways the industrial nursing situation was brought under review. This survey, as complete as it could be under the circumstances, estimated that approximately 1,000 nurses were employed in various industrial fields. Though not by any means all State-registered, this group of assorted nursing grades was found to be providing a pioneer Industrial Nursing Service. On this foundation has been built a structure of no mean proportions.

Some amusing discoveries made during this survey point to a wide variation in the standard of service then available. Evidently believing in the principle of " a penny plain and twopence coloured ", a humble boilerman was found to be charging 2d. for a dry dresssing and 6d. for a hot fomentation to any patient who cared to come to his dug-out for such attention. He filled a definite need and did his best. Amusing also were some of the efforts to encourage employers to establish an industrial nursing service for the first time. An instance comes to mind of a colliery in a South Wales mining valley where the Managing Director was persuaded to develop such a service if the miners would co-operate. Because no District Nursing Association was available in the neighbourhood, it was suggested that a nurse could combine the work of an industrial and district nurse as an experiment. When the question of expense was discussed, it was found that the miners already agreed to several deductions from their weekly pay packet and one item of 1d. a week was willingly given for the upkeep of the Brass Band. When somewhat diffidently a suggestion was made to the men's representatives that perhaps the penny could be split and a half-penny devoted to the provision of a community nursing service, it gained no support and the Brass Band won.

Reference has already been made to the first general meeting called in 1932 by the Public Health Section of the College of Nursing and attended by thirty industrial nurses. Two resolutions were passed at this meeting: first that industrial nurses should be encouraged to join the Public Health Section of the College of Nursing and second that a special training in industrial nursing should be arranged for new entrants to the service. The following year both requests were granted by the Council and the industrial nurse could now be considered as stepping on to the first rung of the ladder towards professional recognition.

In 1934 the first course of training was offered by the Education Department of the College of Nursing in conjunction with Bedford College for Women, Regent's Park, London, N.W.1. It covered an academic year and Miss D. A. Pemberton, S.R.N., later to be Sister-in-Charge, Boots the Chemists, Nottingham, was the only student that year. In a foreword to the Prospectus to this Course Mr. Ernest Bevin, then General Secretary of the Transport and General Workers Union, wrote: " It is particularly encouraging to know that the College of Nursing is introducing a course of study for an Industrial Nursing Certificate and I have read the syllabus with great interest. The constantly changing character of industry calls for specialised study and treatment; each industry has its own peculiar effect upon the physique, whilst in the passing into a chemical age, involving the use of a wide variety of chemical processes, demands that both the medical and nursing professions should become what one might term a 'lookout' brigade. The operation of a particular machine or the use of a special chemical process may produce entirely fresh physical effects. The establishment of this Certificate represents an appreciation of the need to place the physical effects of industry into a special and enlightened category. A tremendous contribution can be made to the health and happiness of a nation by placing at the disposal of productive industry an understanding branch of the medical and nursing profession thereby securing the health of the workpeople." Other encouraging messages were also included in the foreword from Mr. Austen Chamberlain, the Minister of Health, and Lord Trent, speaking for the Government and Industry respectively.

At first two courses were arranged: (A) a whole time course intended for general trained nurses who wished to enter the field of industrial nursing, and (B) a part-time course intended for those already employed in a nursing capacity in industry. The subjects covered by lectures and discussions were: The Health of the Industrial Worker, The Nursing Service in Industry, Social Conditions, The Modern Industrial

System and Psychology. Practical experience in different types of factories was an important feature of Course A.

The fees for Course (A):   College of Nursing Members

                                               30 gns.

                Non-members   45 gns.

       Course (B):   College of Nursing Members

                                               6 gns.

                Non-members   9 gns.

A qualifying certificate was awarded only to candidates who were successful in Course A.

In 1935 a Department of Industrial Hygiene and Medicine at Birmingham University, directed by Dr. Howard Collier, M.C., M.D.(Edin.), Ch.B., was established. One of the objects was " to give facilities for the systematic and advanced teaching for medical practitioners, industrial nurses and welfare workers ". A cordial relationship was soon established between this Department and the College of Nursing, who nominated the writer to serve on the Advisory Board to the University, and the first post-certificate course took place. This was designed to meet the needs of nurses and welfare workers already engaged in industry. It was logical that this should be arranged in an industrial centre such as Birmingham where large numbers of nurses were already employed.

Two letters of interest appeared in *The Times* about this time and to nurses it is a matter for deep gratitude that they were signed by Sir Arthur Stanley, then Chairman of the Council of the College of Nursing. Sir Arthur's sympathy and understanding of the aspirations of industrial nurses prompted him to express, on their behalf, faith in the vision opening before them in the new industrial health service. They are as follows:

To the Editor of The Times. September 14th, 1935.
Sir,
Mr. Hyde's letter published in *The Times* of September 10th is welcomed because it points out how little is known about the

measures which are being introduced to safeguard the health of the worker in industry.

Mr Hyde refers to the work of the Advisory Medical Committee of the Industrial Welfare Society, of which he is Director, and to the recent establishment of the Department of Industrial Hygiene and Medicine at the University of Birmingham, also to the work of the Industrial Health Research Board. It may be of interest to your readers to know, however, that, in order to strengthen the medical side of the work, the College of Nursing have had the question of special training for nurses in preventive methods under consideration for some time past.

The ever widening effect of economic and sociological factors on the prevention of disease has created the need for a woman well trained in nursing procedures and at the same time sympathetic to the special requirements of the employee. In this respect it has been proved that the influence for good which a suitably trained nurse can exert in a factory is unlimited. Under the direction of a medical officer, she is in close touch with the workers. She assists them in times of accident or illness; she is present at their period-ical medical inspections, and she is in a position to give individual and skilled advice on matters of personal hygiene and general health. Last year courses of training were inaugurated by the Council of the College of Nursing for nurses intending to take up work in factories or business houses and for those already employed in industry. The syllabus was drawn up after consulta-tions with medical men and others closely connected with the industrial problems. These courses are to be repeated in the autumn.

The recent development of industry seems to pave the way for an extension of nursing service, particularly among the smaller factories, unable to employ a whole-time medical officer. It appears that the only way to provide this new nursing service is to promote co-operation between closely situated factories in certain areas.

So important does the council of the College consider this new branch of nursing work to be that they have appointed two nurse representatives to attend a conference arranged by the Industrial Welfare Society which begins at Balliol College, Oxford, tomorrow.   I am, Sir, your obedient servant,

ARTHUR STANLEY, Chairman of
The Council of the College of Nursing,
Henrietta Street, W.1.

A little later the following letter appeared:

11th September, 1936.

To the Editor of The Times.

Sir,

Some of your readers may possibly remember two letters published in your columns in September 1935, one by Mr. Robert Hyde, Director of the Industrial Welfare Society and the other by me referring to industrial doctors and to trained nurses in factories respectively.

During the intervening months the field of industry has widened considerably and with this progress is an increasing recognition for the need for supervision of the health of the employees in factories and business houses, for in those places, where schemes have already been developed, the benefit both to the employer and employee is apparent. It is not possible, however, for every firm to employ a doctor and a nurse, therefore greater responsibility is placed on the nurse working alone. The scope of the latter's work is being enlarged, and in addition to the treatment of accidents and minor injuries she is required to advise in a general educational capacity where health is concerned. Where processes involve special risk or strain she may be needed to carry out special treatment or investigation, under medical supervision, for which some knowledge of preventive medicine is required.

That a special training for the work is necessary must be apparent to all who are familiar with the diverse industries of this country. For the past two years the Council of the College of Nursing have endeavoured to provide courses of Instruction for the adequate equipment of nurses in this important and responsible work and courses have been arranged; one for nurses desirous of taking up the work for the first time, the other for those already employed in industry.

At present the number of nurses participating is small for the following reasons: (*a*) the expense involved in taking the course, and (*b*) the salary offered being unlikely to compensate the nurse for the expenditure on the additional training. A few firms have generously offered bursaries and scholarships but more help in this direction is needed. Further, if the woman of education and ability is to be attracted to this important work a salary enabling her to maintain a suitable standard of living should be offered and at least two weeks' continuous holiday each year allowed. She will thus be more able to carry out the principles of healthy living which she is endeavouring to teach.

Sickness invariably leads to serious financial loss not only to employees but to the nation; a more efficient staff in the medical department of firms should do much to reduce this. We should be grateful therefore if the attention of your readers is again directed to a matter which should be the concern of all progressive employers.

I am, Sir, your obedient servant,

ARTHUR STANLEY,

Chairman of Council,

The College of Nursing, Henrietta Street, W.1.

In order to bring these efforts to the notice of individual employers a copy of Sir Arthur's letter was sent by the Council of the College to 2,957 chairmen of industrial firms and 349 Industrial Medical Officers.

The need for money for educational purposes soon became apparent and the nurses themselves arranged a sale at the College of Nursing, realising £47. A scholarship for 38 guineas and a bursary of 6 guineas for the part-time course was offered at once to members of the College from this fund, which has grown considerably over the years and is now generously subscribed to by industry and other interested friends.

The Congress of the International Council of Nurses in 1937 in London has already been referred to. At it the writer gave a paper on " The Place of the Industrial Nurse in Great Britain." The subject aroused considerable interest because few countries were contemplating such a service at that time, and it was then accepted internationally that England was the first country to employ an industrial nurse and that Philippa Flowerday was her name.

The introduction of the Factories Bill in 1937 gave scope for industrial nurses to use their professional machinery in an attempt to influence the proposed legislation. When the Bill was before Parliament in the Committee stage special efforts were made by the College of Nursing to have it amended so that where an ambulance room is provided (in accordance with special regulations and orders) the person in charge should be a State-registered nurse. Officers of the Public Health Section were in attendance at the House during the Committee stage to advise those Members of Parliament who were helping the nurses in their endeavour. These efforts were not entirely successful and as the law stands today the person in charge of the ambulance room is required to be " a qualified nurse or other person trained in first aid ". This loophole makes it possible for lay men and women to be in charge of an ambulance room, but although qualified in the elements of first aid, they cannot be considered to be trained in those principles of the prevention of disease and promotion of health which are essential for the wider interpretation of industrial nursing.

In their campaign the College secured the active support of the National Council of Women and the British Association of Labour Legislation. Questions were asked in Parliament and much help from certain members in the House of Commons and the House of Lords, though unavailing, was given to amend the Bill according to the desire of the nurses. A successful open meeting of nurses under the chairmanship of Miss Margery Fry was held in London on April 7, 1937, which showed conclusively that industrial nurses were now aware of their opportunities, through professional organisation, to influence legislation and the development of their work.

In another direction, about the same time, the Industrial Nurses Sub-Committee of the Public Health Section presented a memorandum to the Royal Commission on Workmen's Compensation in which was the following recommendation: " That the employment of State-registered nurses in factory first-aid departments and ambulance rooms should be more widely extended under statutory orders."

8

Industrial Nursing Organisation (cont.)
The Second World War

WHEN the course of training in industrial nursing offered by the Royal College of Nursing had been established for a few years the thunder clouds of Munich began to gather on the horizon. They brought with them the widely though unwillingly accepted realization that war was imminent and that consequently industrial nurses would be in great demand to help maintain manpower for war work.

Without delay a deputation from the Royal College led by the President, Miss B. Monk, C.B.E., R.R.C., waited upon the Factory Department of the Home Office and offered all the facilities available through their organisation for the recruitment, training and placing of industrial nurses. It is a pleasure to place on record that the deputation was received by the late Dr. J. C. Bridge, C.B.E., F.R.C.S., M.R.C.P., Chief Medical Officer, Factory Department of the Home Office, who by his encouragement and never failing practical help had done so much to guide the early training for this new branch of public health nursing and its subsequent development. To Dr. S. A. Henry, M.A., M.D., D.P.H. (Cantab.) of the same department, appreciation is also expressed for his untiring work on behalf of the industrial nursing students. As a result of these discussions the Royal College was asked to continue the courses for industrial nurses already in existence and to hasten the output of students. Unfortunately it was therefore necessary to shorten the period of study. The arrangements for these courses were in the hands of the Education Department of the Royal College, the tutors being Miss Margaret McEwan, S.R.N., D.N., and Miss F. E. Ingle, S.R.N.

At this time the full-time course which was given at the Royal College covered six months, but later it was reduced to three months. Later still at a request from the Ministry of Labour for an even shorter course, one of six weeks was offered, though students following these lectures were not able to take the examination leading to the industrial nursing certificate of the Royal College. In 1940, to meet the need of those State-registered nurses already in Industry who were unable to leave their work to take the full-time course, a correspondence course was arranged by the College. Students were able to sit for the qualifying examination if they had been employed full time in industry for at least two years. This course was discontinued in 1945.

The transference of the Factory Department of the Home Office to the Ministry of Labour and National Service in 1940 was an important event in the history of industrial nursing.

Appropriate legislation soon followed the appointment of Mr. Ernest Bevin, and Statutory Rules and Orders 1940 No. 1325 was issued. It read as follows:

STATUTORY RULES AND ORDERS
1940 No. 1325

EMERGENCY POWERS (DEFENCE)
Factories (Medical and Welfare Services)

The Factories (Medical and Welfare Services) Order, 1940 Dated July 16, 1940, made by the Minister of Labour and National Service under Regulation 60 of the Defence (General) Regulation, 1939.

In pursuance of the powers conferred on him by Regulation 60 of the Defence (General) Regulations, 1939(a), and of all other powers enabling him in that behalf, the Minister of Labour and National Service (hereinafter referred to as "the Minister") hereby makes the following Orders:

1. The occupier of any factory in which is carried on the manufacture or repair of any munitions of war or of any materials, parts or tools required for such manufacture or repair, or any work on behalf of the Crown shall, if so directed on behalf of the Minister by the Chief Inspector of Factories or by any other Inspector of Factories expressly authorised by the Minister to give directions under the Order, make arrangements to the satisfaction of the Inspector by way of the whole or part-time employment of such numbers of medical practitioners, nurses and supervisory officers as the Inspector may specify, for one or more of the following services, namely:
   (a) medical supervision of persons employed in the factory in the aforesaid manufacture, repair or work,
   (b) nursing and first-aid services for such persons.
   (c) supervision of the welfare of such persons.

2. This Order may be cited as the Factories (Medical and Welfare Services) Order, 1940, and shall come into force on the date hereof.

Signed by Order of the Minister of Labour and National Service this sixteenth day of July, 1940.

(Signed)   T. W. PHILLIPS,
Secretary of the Ministry of
Labour and National Service.

Mr. Bevin received a deputation from the Royal College of Nursing in order to discuss with them certain aspects of industrial nursing including the professional aspect of the nurse's position in Industry and the conditions under which she works, methods of recruitment to the Service and appointment to factories, and the amendment of Statutory Rules and Order 1940 No. 1325 emergency powers (Defence) Factories (Medical and Welfare Services) to include a definition of the term "Nursing Service". The Royal College pressed that this "Nursing Service" should be based on the employment of State-registered nurses responsible to a Medical Officer.

A new era was now dawning for the industrial nurse. The deep and sympathetic understanding and practical help so readily given by Mr. Bevin brought ministerial recognition which inspired a redoubling of effort, and, acceding to his request for training large numbers of industrial nurses, the Royal College set once more to the task. With characteristic directness Mr. Bevin enquired about the cost to the nurse of post-certificate education and there was consequently arranged through his Ministry a system of training grants for this purpose. The following is the announcement of the financial arrangements issued.

MINISTRY OF LABOUR AND NATIONAL SERVICE INDUSTRIAL NURSES
Special Course of Instruction

The rapid expansion of the National effort has greatly enhanced the importance of the work of nurses in factories and it is desired to increase the number of trained nurses with special qualifications for posts as industrial nurses.

The work which nurses are required to do in factories differs in many respects from what they are required to do in hospitals and private practice, and it is desirable that nurses intending to take employment in factories should receive some special training for the work they are to undertake.

The course of training arranged by the Royal College of Nursing and previously taken by nurses intending to enter industry extended over six and twelve months, but this was reduced to three months at the outbreak of war.

To meet the present need, a short intensive course of instruction has been arranged in collaboration with the Royal College of Nursing and with various employers having medical supervision and well-established first-aid ambulance arrangements in their factories.

This leaflet relates to the procedure and facilities afforded in the case of this special intensive course of instruction.

Qualifications

The course will be open to women and men who have taken up nursing as a profession, have received the usual professional training and are either registered or eligible for registration on the General Part of the Register. It is essential that candidates should possess qualities which will enable them to gain readily the confidence both of employers and of work-people. Candidates under the age of 27 years would not normally be regarded as suitable and they should, of course, be physically fit to undertake the work. Candidates will not normally be accepted if they possess qualifications in, or experience of types of nursing (and midwifery) where the supply of personnel is particularly short. Applications will not be considered from women and men who are employed in a senior post.

Application by and Selection of Candidates
Selection of candidates to undergo the course of instruction will be carried out by a Selection Board appointed by the Minister of Labour and National Service.

Applications must be made on a form which can be obtained from the Ministry of Labour and National Service (A.7), St. James's Square, London, S.W.1. or from the Royal College of Nursing, Henrietta Place, Cavendish Square, London, W.1. Completed forms must be returned to the Ministry of Labour and National Service at the address given above.

No candidates will be selected by the Board for admission to the course except after a personal interview before the Board.

Course of Instruction
The course will last for approximately six weeks, part of which will be spent by students in factories selected under arrangements made by the Ministry in conjunction with the Royal College of Nursing, where they will receive practical training in the work. Attendance at the course of instruction will not entitle a student to any certificate of proficiency.

Financial Arrangements
In the case of candidates selected by the Board under the scheme, the fees for the course will be paid by the Ministry on behalf of the student. Such candidates would also be paid an allowance on the following scales:

1. While attending at the instructional centre if within daily travelling distance of student's home ...... 26s. per week. Reasonable daily travelling expenses to and from the centre may be allowed when it is necessary to travel more than two miles each way.

2. While attending at the centre where the student has to live
away from home .... 50s. per week.
No special allowance will be made in respect of the cost (if any)
incurred by the student in obtaining books required for the
course.

Third-class railway fares will be refunded to candidates summoned
to attend for interview by the Selection Board.
Travelling expenses, third class, may be paid to students from
home to the place of instruction, and, at the end of the course, to
the place of employment or home. Travelling expenses to the
place where the practical instruction is given may also be paid.

General
Persons accepted for instruction will be expected to complete
the course and those who for any reason fail to do so may be
required to refund the expenses incurred on their behalf.
Acceptance for a course does not imply any guarantee of employment as an industrial nurse but every effort will be made by the
Ministry of Labour and National Service to place persons who
complete the course in posts where their training will be utilised.

Ministry of Labour and National Service,
8 St. James's Square, London, S.W.1.

P.L. 140/1943.   September, 1943.

It should be mentioned that the Royal College of Nursing
had provided, at considerable strain on its funds, the finance
for all the industrial training courses and had been dealing with
the multitudinous problems concerning the nursing profession which arose out of the expansion of the Industrial
Nursing Service and those difficulties which resulted from the
Control of Engagement Order, registration of nurses and
other war time regulations.

Requests for training began to come from nurses in industrial centres outside London where the need was urgent
and pressing. As a result of an approach to the Nuffield Provincial Hospitals Trust for assistance in extending training
through the Provincial universities, a grant of £1,885 was
given to the Royal College and training was subsequently

arranged at the Universities of Glasgow, Cardiff, Bristol, Leeds, Belfast and Liverpool and at University College, Nottingham. An appeal to industry brought further funds for assisting these educational developments in industrial nursing. Taking these courses outside London were 175 students. Running concurrently were facilities for a Correspondence Course and tribute is here paid to many nurses who, bearing the heat and burden of the day, still found time to study and prepare themselves for the examination for the industrial nursing certificate of the Royal College.

An amusing story illustrating the busy lives which industrial nurses were leading while following their industrial nursing training course can be recalled. An industrial nursing student, finding, as so many of them did, that the industrial and economic structure of the country was the subject needing greater concentration than other sections of the syllabus, thought she would obtain first-hand information about labour organisation by questioning the working man himself. The day of her examination had come and she was at the railway station on her way to sit for this particular paper. Choosing her compartment with care where a group of men were already seated, at the right moment she asked, " What can you tell me about Trade Unions? " and from the oldest man in the corner came the reply, " Miss, I don't 'old wi' 'em! "

The war effort was now gathering momentum and nurses were in tremendous demand. As evidence of the power of broadcasting it is of interest to record that when the writer spoke in the Home Service of the B.B.C. on " One more opportunity for Women " there was a response by telephone to the Royal College of Nursing within twenty minutes of the broadcast and volunteers to the Service continued to flow in steadily. Industrial nursing had become a popular field of national service.

Caxton Hall, Westminster, was the scene of an impressive Conference on Industrial Health in 1943 which was convened by the Ministry of Labour and National Service. Its purpose was to emphasise the importance of industrial health and to elicit further suggestions for promoting it. The proceedings included speeches by Ministers, papers by a number of Government and other experts and contributions from those attending. Constructive plans were put forward by Mrs. A. L. Reeve, S.R.N. and Miss J. M. Tolfree, S.R.N. both of whom at that time were industrial students at the Royal College of Nursing. Their contributions to the discussion may be summarised as follows:

> The war, with its need for increased production and at the same time its demand for more and more man-power for the Armed Forces, has shown the importance of maintaining the health of the workers. Many managements have been led to realise the advantage, both to the workers and in the interests of production, of the introduction of works surgeries and doctors available for industry and, just as the engineers, by breaking down their jobs, have been able to train housewives to do the work formerly done by highly skilled technicians, so must the doctors accept this principle of dilution in their work. Suitably trained nurses are the most obvious people to meet this need.
>
> Very little provision has been made so far for the special training of Industrial Medical Officers, but a three months' intensive course is available for nurses wishing to prepare themselves for this special branch of work, also a six weeks' course subsidised by the Ministry of Labour. In London and other industrial centres, the Royal College of Nursing has organised this training, in which the basic principles of industrial health are taught, against the background of an understanding of labour relations, in addition to practical work in factories and public health organisations concerned with industrial problems. This course is turning out a considerable number of nurses anxious to play their full part in the fight for health in the factories. As in all preventive medicine, the work of the nurse in industry will be largely educative; such matters as health education, close observation of working conditions, and the understanding of women's problems, that form such an important contribution to war-time health questions, are all subjects with which she is particularly suited to deal.

At present there are several thousand nurses working in industry, many of them pioneers who have helped to build up first-class health units in individual factories, but the duties they are called upon to perform are as diverse as their qualifications and training. In a certain factory engaged in light industry, with no special hazards and employing only 150 workers, there are three full-time trained nurses, whereas other groups of industrial workers are entirely without medical and nursing supervision. Legitimate criticism has been aroused, in the acute shortage of nurses that war precipitates, as to whether all these nurses in industry are being put to their fullest use, or whether they should not be directed back into the grossly understaffed hospitals. Yet it is true that an efficient health service at the point of production will prevent many cases of illness or accident ever requiring hospital treatment. The nurses themselves may feel that preventive medicine is unreal and less urgent than the demands of actual patients in hospital clamouring for treatment and attention. The hospital training provides too little link-up between the clinical and social aspects of disease.

What seems to be needed, therefore, is a planned distribution of these nurses, who have some special training in industrial health. The Government are committed to the introduction of a National Medical Service in some form or another and it may be assumed that the establishment of an Industrial Medical Service would be a part of any such scheme. Only by taking the health of the worker out of the hands of the individual employers and making it a public concern can the wise and economic use of the forces available be achieved.

The following suggestions are put forward for consideration in any scheme to be formulated:

1. Greater pressure should be brought to bear by the Government upon factory managements to provide reasonable, well-equipped works surgeries, under nursing control. Definite standards should be laid down as to what is considered necessary. Small factories should be grouped into units, sharing the facilities available.

2. Nurses engaged in industry should have special industrial training and should be appointed by an authority qualified to judge their ability. A register of those qualified should be kept and they could be registered as mobile and immobile.

3. All nurses should be required to take revision classes periodically and these might be arranged regionally by the Royal College of Nursing. Special leave should be granted for this purpose.

4. A panel of inspectors should be organised to visit all works surgeries at intervals to ensure that the standard of treatment, equipment, and general efficiency is maintained. Reports of these inspections should be kept at a central office which could also issue instructions to those health departments which fell short of the required standards. The inspectors should be industrially trained nurses of experience.

5. Medical records should be inspected regularly and a précis forwarded to the central authority. If standard methods of record-keeping were introduced the collection of statistics would prove very valuable, both in shedding light on weak points in industry in general and on individual factories in particular.

6. Greater scope for treatment in works surgeries, particularly where a medical officer is appointed, should be permitted and encouraged.

7. Opportunities should be given for exchange of views and experience among nurses engaged in different factories.

The problem of the Health of the worker is of paramount importance and any plan formulated should be regarded as an essential part of the war effort and not only as a scheme for post-war reconstruction. Its speedy adoption is essential if the health of the workers, with its influence on production, is to be maintained and improved to enable them to shoulder the increasing demands that will inevitably fall on them before victory is achieved.

The many and complex problems with which the Royal College of Nursing was concerned during the rapid development of industrial nursing in the early days of the war prompted the Council to set up an advisory committee, its terms of reference being:

"To act in an advisory capacity on matters dealing with industrial nursing."

The members of the Committee were:

Miss D. C. Coode, S.R.N., Chairman of Council, Royal College of Nursing.

Miss D. M. Smith, S.R.N., Deputy Chairman of Council, who was Chairman of the Advisory Committee.

Miss I. H. Charley, S.R.N., Chairman, Public Health Section, Royal College of Nursing.

Miss D. Pemberton, S.R.N., Sister-in-Charge, Boots the Chemists.

Miss A. A. Saville, S.R.N., Women's Personnel Officer, Electrolux Ltd.

Air Vice-Marshal Sir David Munro, K.C.B., C.I.E., M.A., LL.D., M.B., Ch.B. (Ed.), F.R.C.S. (Ed.), Chief Medical Officer, Ministry of Supply.

Sir Wilson Jameson, K.C.B., M.A., M.D., LL.D., F.R.C.P., Dean, London School of Hygiene and Tropical Medicine.

Dr. W. D. Jenkins, M.R.C.S., L.R.C.P., Chief Medical Officer, South Metropolitan Gas Company.

Miss Mary Jones, O.B.E., A.R.R.C., M.A., S.R.N., Matron, Liverpool Royal Infirmary.

Dr. (now Professor) R. E. Lane, M.B., B.S., F.R.C.P., Medical Officer, Chloride Electricity Co. Ltd.

Dr. Donald Stewart, M.D., F.R.C.P. (Ed.), Chief Medical Officer, Austin Motor Co. Ltd., Birmingham.

Dr. S. A. Henry, M.A., M.D., D.P.H.(Cantab.), Factory Department, Ministry of Labour and National Service.

Miss F. Taylor, S.R.N., D.N. (University of London), Sister Tutor, Guy's Hospital.

Miss M. Houghton, S.R.N., D.N. (University of London), Sister Tutor, University College Hospital.

Miss P. Darbyshire, S.R.N., Matron-in-Chief, Trained Nurses' Department, British Red Cross Society.

Miss G. Hillyers, S.R.N., Matron, St. Thomas's Hospital.

The Committee confined its attention chiefly to the scope and duties of the industrial nurse and the advice which was available from such a distinguished group of medical and nursing authorities did much to lay the firm foundations on which the new service has grown.

By October 1942 the nurses themselves were learning the value of professional organisation as a means through which their opinion could be voiced for the shaping of their new service and at a large meeting of industrial nurses called by the

Royal College of Nursing, a resolution was passed, the principles of which were endorsed by the Advisory Committee and incorporated in the policy of the Royal College as it concerned industrial nursing.

The resolution was as follows:

That:

(a) The time has come to clarify the relative functions and status of the Industrial Nurse and Welfare Supervisor.

(b) Industrial nursing is a branch of public health nursing and in all aspects of the nurse's work the emphasis should be paid on the prevention of disease and the promotion of health.

(c) Industrial health is a function of personnel management.

(d) The industrial nurse is responsible to the medical officer whether he is employed full time or part time. If no medical officer is employed the nurse is responsible to the managing director or his appointed deputy.

(e) If a welfare supervisor and an industrial nurse are employed both shall have equal status and be paid comparable salaries.

(f) In all factories employing up to 1,000 (500 for heavy industries) the post of nurse and welfare supervisor can be combined. A nurse holding a combined post should have the Industrial Nursing Certificate together with the appropriate welfare training.

(g) In the case of the smaller factory where the employment of a State-registered nurse is uneconomical a system of grouping is necessary. Under this scheme factories in an area can with advantage, be grouped and one nurse qualified as under paragraph (f) be employed by the group.

(h) Where the industrial organisation is such that the posts cannot be combined, it is considered that the functions of the industrial nurse should include:

    i. pre-employment examination and interviews.

    ii. health services—accident and industrial disease hazards.

    iii. auxiliary health service, e.g. dental, optical, chiropody, ray-therapy, etc.

    iv. health education.

    v. medical records and reports.

vi. medical social service including:
- (a) rehabilitation of the injured worker.
- (b) co-operation with community health services.
- (c) sick visiting.
- (d) convalescent care.

Industrial Nursing Training at Birmingham Accident Hospital.

In the first report of the Birmingham Accident Hospital and Rehabilitation Centre it is recorded that on April 1, 1941, the Provisional Board of the Hospital took over the building and equipment of the Queen's Hospital, Birmingham, which ceased to exist as a general hospital. Certain of the surgical, nursing and administrative staff were transferred from the Queen's Hospital to the new Hospital. Thus was established in Birmingham the first specialised hospital devoted entirely to the treatment and rehabilitation of men and women injured through accident.

The middle of the war might be thought to be an unsuitable time for establishing a new hospital; it was soon apparent, however, that the need for a hospital specialising in the treatment of accidents was greater in time of war than in peace time. During the previous two years the number of industrial injuries in the Birmingham area requiring treatment at hospitals had increased by at least 40 per cent, the total being well over 100,000 per annum. Such a figure represents an incalculable loss to the nation's man-power through lost time with consequent serious upset of production and lowered output, nor can the consequent suffering be measured. Therefore the importance of specialised treatment for injured persons and their return to maximum activity as soon as possible had never been greater than at that time. Geographically the hospital was well situated. It was close to the centre of the city and was therefore particularly suitable for outpatients. An accident hospital must of necessity have a large and well-organised out-patient department and special provisions must be made for dealing with patients quickly.

The report pointed out that with the war there had been a great increase in the demand for trained nurses for industry. In fact the demand in the Midlands frequently exceeded the supply. Moreover, industrial nursing presented problems not covered in ordinary general training. The Board had prepared a scheme for training State-registered nurses in industrial nursing and it was expected that Birmingham University would grant a Certificate in Industrial Nursing. It would enable factories and other business organisations to secure the services of highly trained nurses as and when required, through a Bureau to be set up at the Hospitals and would ensure that present industrial nursing staff was kept in touch with modern methods. An experimental course had been running during the past six months and had been appreciated by the students.

The establishment of a medical department in the Ministry of Supply bringing several hundred nurses within the government—owned or—controlled factories into one service called for the appointment of a Chief Nursing Officer and Miss F. Clare Sykes, M.B.E., S.R.N., S.C.M., D.N., Ind. Nursing Cert., was appointed in 1942. In *The Proceedings of the Ninth International Congress of Industrial Medicine, London* 1948. *Section C. Session 11—The Administration of an Industrial Nursing Service*, Miss Sykes described the development of her work in the Ministry of Supply and it seems appropriate to quote extracts here in her own words. She said:

The Ministry of Supply was created in 1939 and its supply and manufacturing sections produced all the munitions of war, guns, shells, bombs, small arms, torpedoes and mines. During the war this Ministry became the largest business unit in Great Britain. It had factories employing 30,000 people at one end of the scale and factories employing a few hundred at the other. ' New Entrants ' poured into these factories, where they would work in contact with hazardous substances, at the rate of hundreds a week. The medical departments began with the work of isolated groups of doctors and nurses who were concerned chiefly with the examination of new entrants and the provision of first aid to the sick and injured; they developed into highly organised centres providing a comprehensive industrial medical service. The medical department team in the larger factories came to include doctors and nurses, first-aid orderlies, dispensers, a physiotherapist, a dentist, a chiropodist and an optician.

In its early period the Ministry of Supply Nursing Service had all the defects characteristic of industrial nursing in the period between the wars. Nurses were recruited sometimes by doctors, but quite as often by factory superintendents, personnel officers, even chief engineers, who were not qualified to evaluate nursing education and experience. None of the nurses so recruited had any previous training or experience in industrial nursing and the great majority of the doctors were likewise without experience in industrial medicine. These isolated groups had no contact with each other and no thought had been given, or professional advice taken, on their conditions of service which were not uniform throughout the whole service. A factor most injurious to their self-respect and to the development of any professional pride in their service was that their professional status, so assured in hospital practice, was ignored in the bewildering world of these munition factories working under inconceivable stress to ' produce at all costs '.

Briefly the lessons to be drawn are, the necessity first to appoint a Chief Medical Officer and a Chief Nursing Officer, so as to ensure that recruitment of staff and development shall be on sound professional lines and to give much thought to conditions of service and status, which should be comparable to those in other professional specialities. In October 1940 Sir David Munro was appointed Chief Medical Officer to be succeeded on his retirement in July 1943 by Dr. Amor. I, myself, was appointed Chief Nursing Officer in December 1942 with the following broad directives:

To advise on nursing complements and grades in Ministry of Supply establishments and on the scope of nursing duties and responsibilities.

To select and recommend recruitment of nursing staff.

To establish and maintain industrial nursing standards and undertake the further education and training for industry of nursing staff.

To be responsible for professional discipline.

To maintain nursing records.

The administrative problem was threefold. We had to instil a a pride in the service and build up morale. We had to teach the principles and practice of industrial nursing; the toxicology of the wide variety of toxic substances which our workers handled and the principles of the control and prevention of their hazards to health and safety; the place of the medical departments in relation to factory organisation and to other community health service. Finally we had to devise administrative procedures to control selection, engagement, transference, promotion and termination of staff appointments and conditions of service. Our results had to be achieved quickly for we were an organisation in being, in the throes of our problems, not an organisation whose administrative lines had been well thought out in times of peace and were projected in tranquillity. Thus from the first, education was placed in the forefront of our policy and the educational function of our supervision was the one we most stressed.

Our efforts to infuse a good service were guided by two basic principles. First the Medical and Nursing Service were to be developed and to function as *One Service* with differing but joint functions and combined in differing proportions according to the needs of each establishment, the doctor/nurse team was regarded as the essential unit of the service. If our industrial health units are to attain the highest efficiency and to function harmoniously, doctors and nurses of equally good calibre must be recruited and given a thorough training in the principles and practice of industrial medicine with, as well as an emphasis on their own, an appreciation of each other's functions.

Our second basic principle was the value of personal contact between the administrative heads of the service and the scattered factory staffs. In the early days of what we came to call the 'Formulative Stage' of the service in distinction to the 'Chaotic Stage' which has preceded it, I spent 75 per cent of my time in the factories and their medical departments, observing, listening, hearing all the criticisms, searching out and weighing the problems and difficulties, enlisting co-operation in finding solutions, or, where that was not attainable, pointers to sound lines of progress. Days in the factory were followed by informal evening conferences with Medical Officers and Sisters. During our third stage, the 'Stage of Implementation' proportionally more time had of course to be spent at Headquarters initiating and revising policies tentatively formulated during those exploratory visits.

Nothing perhaps did more to encourage keenness than the knowledge individual members of staff thus gained that they were moulding the service. Of first importance during the constructive period of an organisation, and even at a much later stage when lines of administration had been clarified, personal contact between the adminstrative officer and factory staffs should not be allowed to lapse.

Indeed it is in the later stages that, if great care is not taken—and here the steadily broadening education programme is most valuable as a positive and creative force—an organisation becomes lifeless. The administrative lines may be sound but yet no living currents flow along them. Administratively an organisation may be chaotic, yet instilled with life and creative ideas. Our desired goal is an orderly organisation which yet nourishes and develops the creative contributions of all its individuals. There is a regrettable tendency for all administrators to become desk-bound, issuers of memoranda rather than living personalities to their staffs, concerned to foster interchange of experience, to widen mental horizons, and what is perhaps most important of all to sound policy making, to stimulate and evoke the interchange of thought and ideas so that each staff member has opportunity to contribute to the life of her organisation.

In any field of administration a most perplexing problem is how to develop over the whole field a uniformly high standard without crushing initiative by rendering staff 'regulation-bound'. Perhaps one pointer to the solution lies here, in the maximum development of the individual within the framework of the organisation, in staff discussions, formal and informal, at all levels; and in the confrontation of the individual as frankly as possible with the problems of the organisation as a whole and inviting his or her contributions to the solution. There is a twofold gain here. Most administrators have had practical experience, but the passage of years causes this to wax a little dim; it may also cause her to draw deductions from it which seem to an increasing restive staff irrelevant to the new circumstances. Much more realistic policies are likely to issue from staff consultations in the formulative stage. The gain to members of staff is that they imbibe, almost without realising it, a training in the analysis and solution of adminstrative problems and techniques.

An educational policy begins with the selection of staff and this is the most important if you accept, as an incentive to good work, the principle of promotion to senior posts from within the Service. Any organisation selects its recruits to as high a standard as circumstances permit. During the war, and to a lesser extent since, in the continuing shortage of nurses, it is easy for a nursing adminstrator to grow discouraged. Industrial nursing at its best demands a good standard of general education, wide professional experience, insight into human and social problems, skill in handling human relations, and a quality of poise and adaptability. We may feel a little cheered, however, to reflect that only a very small proportion of our intake can achieve senior posts in the factories and of those only a fraction will eventually become industrial nurse tutors and administrators. Therefore if a year's intake into a single service yields only a small percentage which can definitely be classed as 'leadership material', there is no cause for despair. In any organisation as a whole the good routine worker has a high importance—the girl who will work pleasantly and dependably in her factory, who is conscientious and teachable. There is such a thing as the good follower as well as the good leader and her value to the organisation is inestimable. When, after analysis of the educational, professional and personal record and after a personal interview with the applicants, one has eliminated those with definite contra-indications to suitability, one finds that one's recruits consist of a very small batch of 'leader potential' and a much larger batch of 'ordinary quality'. Amongst the latter, closer contact reveals fascinating mixtures of strengths and weaknesses in each individual and it is the task of supervision, as it is that of the tutor with her students, to develop each staff member, to use her capabilities to the full and to strengthen the weaknesses, to enlarge her range without overstraining her.

The answer to the question 'who should select and by what methods?' must partly depend on the Company's or Department's staff selection procedures. The Selection Board should, however, always include an experienced industrial nurse and senior sister in charge of staff; nor should a Medical Officer be regarded as a substitute for her. A good Selection Board is one which includes a Medical Officer who has successfully practised industrial medicine at factory level and been directly responsible for the staff of a factory medical department, an industrial nursing sister and at least one lay member. On methods of selection, I would like to see further investigations. We in this country have perhaps been rather conservative, not quite convinced of the validity of any tests for those traits of temperament and personality so important in industrial nursing. While it is advisable for the Chief Nursing Administrator to be responsible for staff recruitment, it is also wise policy to allow her discretion to delegate this; she will be wise at once to retain in her own hands this power of delegation but to use it as often as she feels it safe to do so. While undoubtedly some have a flair for choosing the right people, good staff selection improves with practice and senior sisters, as well as Medical Officers, should be encouraged to use their judgment upon it.

. . . *The Ministry of Supply Nursing Service Bulletin*, edited by the Chief Nursing Officer, is issued bi-monthly to all nursing staffs. It is at once a link between staffs, a vehicle of discussion of matters of current interest, and an information service. We publish in it articles by outside authorities, by our own Medical Officers and Sisters, staff members and safety officers, production managers, research and work chemists, etc. on industrial medicine and nursing, occupational hazards, accident prevention and so on. We include also abstracts and digests on such subjects from current journals, book reviews, and articles on social service and education.

Group education is both internal and external. Any large and scattered service requires internal staff courses and conferences. It is usual for Ministry of Supply internal staff courses to be held in the spring and autumn—four courses each with not more than twenty students, at one of our larger factories. Such courses last three or three and a half days. Compilation of each syllabus is based on staff suggestions, often put forward through Senior Sisters' conferences. Lectures and demonstrations and discussions are given and led both by outside experts and by our own medical officers, sisters and factory administrators. Much time is given to discussion and opportunities for the supervised practice of techniques. Opportunity is also given to study processes and health hazards in other industries; for example, a course centred on a Staffordshire factory would include lectures on the pottery industry of that area and a visit to a pottery. Such courses, bringing our sisters and nurses into social and professional contact with each other and with the heads of the Medical and Nursing Service, have done much to foster a Service spirit as well as to quicken interest and improve performance.

But special care must also be taken in a large organisation not to become self-contained, and to encourage keeping in touch with professional colleagues in other organisations. We therefore encourage attendance at Refresher Courses and Study Days organised by the Universities and by the Royal College of Nursing and travelling and subsistence allowance are granted for such attendance.

It is also important to give individual tuition and systematically to widen individual experience. Sisters, for instance, have been sent individually for tuition to the Industrial Ophthalmic Unit of the Royal Arsenal, to the Medical Department of the Electric Chloride Company, and the Birmingham Accident Hospital; to a radiological unit at Cambridge, and to selected hospitals for courses in x-ray work. Interchange is also being arranged between Sisters from one of our factories in the north-west and Sisters from the Mersey Docks and Harbour Board Medical Service. Such interchanges guard at once against staleness and complacency.

From this description it can be seen that from the chaos which was evident in the early days of Industrial Nursing in the Ministry of Supply, there emerged a nursing service of no mean proportions.

All this time literature on industrial nursing was conspicuous by its absence until *A Handbook for Industrial Nurses* by Marion M. West, S.R.N., S.C.M., appeared in 1941. This volume was the only textbook for some time and remains a standard work of reference. A second edition appeared in 1949. Air Vice-Marshal Sir David Munro, K.C.B., Chief Medical Officer to the Ministry of Supply, in a foreword to this book, said: " The gate is open for the industrial nurse to enter on a new kind of professional career. But for this she needs training. . . . It is my earnest hope that this new branch of nursing will receive the recognition it deserves, both in status and remuneration."

In 1944 *Industrial Nursing. Its Aims and Practice* by Mrs. A. B. Dowson-Weisskopf, S.R.N., Ind. Nursing Cert., was published. Industrial nursing literature remained an urgent need during these days and although isolated articles or series of articles appeared in the nursing press little attention was given to the subject. This was, no doubt, due to the paper shortage situation during the war and also the pre-occupation of those who, although realising the lack of reading material, were unable to devote time to its production. In 1944, however, the *British Journal of Physical Medicine* reserved space in each issue for a special feature under the title " For the Industrial Nurse ". This was edited by Miss Marion M. West, S.R.N., S.C.M., and has been a useful forum through which current matters of concern to the industrial nurse have been brought to their notice and discussed. A development in 1947 through the Industrial Nurses' Discussion Group in the Public Health Section of the London Branch of the Royal College of Nursing was the publication of a News Letter which served as a link between the members of the group and others who were interested.

When Mr. Ernest Bevin announced that he was setting up a Factory Welfare Advisory Board, its terms of reference being " to develop to the fullest extent the safety, health and welfare arrangements inside the factories and the billeting, communal feeding and welfare arrangements outside the factories ", Miss Clare Sykes was appointed to the Board on the nomination of the Royal College of Nursing and the profession was much gratified that its new contribution to industrial health and welfare had received ministerial recognition.

Under the Chairmanship of Lady Cynthia Colville, D.C.V.O., J.P., a Central Consultative Committee was established bringing together all the voluntary associations having a contribution to make to the well-being of industrial workers. Groups dealing with health, juvenile needs, recreational facilities, professional requirements and general matters were established. The Royal College of Nursing was represented on those groups considering health and professional requirements.

The duties of the industrial nurse, particularly in relation to other welfare officers employed in the factory, were much debated by the nurses at this time. In order to come to a satisfactory conclusion, realising that the work was constantly developing to meet the expanding needs of industry and to guide the newcomers to the Service, certain suggestions were made and a summary was published by the Royal College of Nursing.

The suggested duties of the industrial nurse were:

1. To be responsible for the general efficiency of the ambulance room and of any other first-aid arrangements in the factory. To assist as may be desirable in supplementary training of any first-aid personnel.

2. To have adequate knowledge of the hazards and various processes of the work in the factory.

3. To undertake first-aid treatment of injury and of sickness and such subsequent treatment as may be ordered by the patient's medical attendant that can adequately be done in the ambulance room.

4. To keep adequate and suitable records of all cases of injury or sickness receiving attention at the ambulance room or elsewhere in the factory.

5. To present to the management at regular intervals a suitable summary of the work done.

6. To organise the best method of presenting those requiring medical examination.

7. To give every assistance in the examination of workers at the factory either by the examining surgeon or other medical officer.

8. To promote the education of the work-people collectively and individually in matters of general and personal hygiene.

9. To co-operate with heads of departments, foremen and the executive personnel.

10. To co-operate with any existing welfare department.

11. To co-operate with canteen management.

12. To assist as may be required in a professional capacity in the A.R.P. services of the factory.

13. To advise all workers returning to work after sickness or injury.

14. To make recommendation to the management regarding facilities for obtaining any special diet which is medically advised.

15. To co-operate with outside health and other social services for the benefit of the workers whether in sickness or in health.

16. To see all workers before they are sent home for any reason of injury or ill health.

17. To co-operate with the Labour Management and Welfare Department in:

    (a) selecting applicants for engagement from the point of view of health.

    (b) regard to pending dismissal for other than disciplinary reasons.

18. To keep suitable confidential records of physical conditions on engagement, providing space for subsequent medical history.

19. To receive notifications of all absentees from the appropriate department and to record the cause, if known.

20. To compile absence figures when no statistical department is already in existence.

21. To visit the homes, circumstances permitting, in order to maintain contact with the sick or injured workers and to notify the District Nursing Association on their behalf.

22. To maintain contact in economic welfare with regard to the disposal of thrift benevolent funds and other contributory schemes.

23. To co-operate with any safety committee.

24. To be responsible where no special department is in existence for the proper use and care of all protective clothing.

N.B. The above duties may vary in detail if there is a factory doctor employed.

Many and varied, however, were the duties which fell to industrial nurses during the war and one nurse remembers with pride a small service which she rendered to Mr. Winston Churchill. In the bowels of the earth, beneath a busy newspaper office in Fleet Street, during the blitz on London, she was privileged to prepare coffee and light meals for him and Lord Beaverbrook as they sheltered from the falling bombs. Often arriving after midnight they would snatch a brief hour's sleep on simple shelter beds covered by the familiar grey A.R.P. blankets. With an inexhaustible capacity for work they would be ready for the next day before the grey dawn was creeping over the horizon and the " All clear " was uttering its melancholy wail.

In a memorandum on Medical Supervision in Factories (Form 327. Nov. 1940) issued by the Factory Department of the Ministry of Labour and National Service is a paragraph on nursing which says: " The efficiency of the first-aid arrangements will be greatly increased by the employment (as is now an increasing practice) of a State-registered nurse (or nurses) or one holding a certificate from a recognised hospital. It is very desirable that the nurse, particularly in large factories, should have received special training in industrial nursing or have had previous experience of such work in factories. The nurse can relieve the Medical Officer of much of the first-aid treatment of injury and sickness in the factory and such subsequent treatment as may be considered desirable to perform in the ambulance room. She would be responsible to him for the general efficiency of the ambulance room and other first-aid arrangements. . . ." " Provided that a fully trained nurse is in charge, additional assistance can in many circumstances be adequately provided by one or more less qualified but suitably trained persons. The nurse's close association with the employees facilitates the Medical Officer's attention being drawn to such cases as require examination, while the value of her presence during any examination of the employees, and assistance in keeping of records, is obvious."

It is impossible in a survey like this to mention all the spheres of influence to which the industrial nurse was introduced during the war years, but an outstanding development initiated by the Ministry of War Transport with the creation of the

Mersey Docks Medical Service, and later a similar service by the Clyde Navigation Trust, should take its rightful place in this history. Chief Nursing Officers were appointed to both these services, Miss M. S. Pinkerton, S.R.N., at Liverpool and Miss M. Macgregor Thomson, S.R.N., at Glasgow.

Two main features in the professional organisation of the of the industrial nurse through the Public Health Section of the Royal College of Nursing at this time were outstanding, both illustrating the serious approach of the nurses to their work. One was the desire of the nurses to organise profession-ally and to improve through education and further training their service to the industry. Another feature was the arrange-ment up and down the country of day or week-end courses of study. The hospitality of industrial firms or the extra-mural departments of Universities, such as Manchester, where Dr. (now Professor) R. E. Lane, M.B., B.S., F.R.C.P., gave great encouragement, was much appreciated and the high attendance at such courses in spite of blackout conditions and much restricted transport facilities testifies to the great desire of the nurses to benefit by an exchange of ideas and professional intercourse. Local branches and Public Health Sections of the Royal College also gave much service and generous hospitality in arranging study courses.

But rapid development brings with it unavoidable problems. The somewhat haphazard growth, varying standards of service and adminstrative difficulties, needed continual vigilance on the part of the Royal College of Nursing. Many of the prob-lems were due to a lack of appreciation of the status of the State-registered nurse in industry, as employers were often unaware of the wider scope of industrial nursing envisaged by the profession. They frequently wanted to restrict her activities to the ambulance room only, failing to appreciate her useful-ness in the wide field of labour relations and welfare.

A code of ethics and scale of salaries was drawn up by the Industrial Nurses Sub-Committee of the Public Health Section of the Royal College and the response indicated the desire of industry to recompense the nurse more generously. There were discussions on service conditions with the Engineering and Allied Employers' National Federation, the Ministry of Supply, the Admiralty, and the Iron and Steel Trades Federation and by degrees better salary scales were accepted voluntarily by employers.

The experience of industrial nurses was brought to bear on the war economy of the country in many ways and when in 1943 a select Committee on National Expenditure was set up by the Goverment, a Committee of women M.P.s, of which Miss Irene Ward was Chairman and Viscountess Davidson an active member, asked for evidence from the Royal College of Nursing, which was gathering together the practical experience of industrial nurses. Such subjects as conditions of employment of women in industry, the provision of facilities for personal hygiene, and the need for medical examination of women before leaving home when called up for national service were discussed. The value of the prompt action taken by this group of women M.P.s on behalf of women in industry, cannot be overestimated.

In the same way the Royal College of Nursing contributed to the deliberations of the Woman Power Committee, the driving force behind the official scheme to make adequate use of women workers in war factories. Miss Irene Ward, M.P., was Chairman of the Committee, other members being Mrs. E. M. Wood, C.B.E. (Hon. Secretary), Miss Eleanor Rathbone, M.P., Miss Dorothy Elliott and Dame Caroline Haslett, D.B.E., who, as President of the Women's Engineering Society and Director of the Electrical Association for Women, was adviser to the Ministry of Labour and National Service on women's training. Largely as a result of the work of this group, free training for women to work in fitting and machine shops was achieved. Before this concession was granted women were obliged to pay for their own training.

The Public Health Section of the Royal College of Nursing presented several memoranda to the Ministry of Labour and National Service during the war, stressing among other things their opinion that industrial nurses had a large part to play in the war production campaign. It was not necessary for the Royal College to emphasise that one of the most serious disorganising factors in industrial life is absence due to illness— not only long and serious illness but the shorter and so-called minor ailments such as the common cold, tonsillitis, boils, headaches, etc. That was well known; but the nurse's part in reducing absenteeism was not always recognised. The need for "follow-up" of all absence due to sickness was also the subject of representation to the Factory Welfare Advisory Board and the part which could be played by the Queen's nurse in the homes of the workers in this respect was emphasised. Largely as a result of these discussions, a confidential circular, dated November 30, 1940, dealing with nursing for transferred war workers was issued by the Ministry of Health.

In the report for the years 1939-1946 of the Ministry of Labour and National Service, the following note appears, indicating that full use was made of District Nursing Associations in providing home nursing care for munition workers.

PROVISION IN RESPECT OF SICKNESS

" The accommodation of workers in lodgings or billets inevitably involved special provision for ' Home nursing' when they were sick. Where necessary, arrangements were made in collaboration with the Health Departments for the worker to be cared for under the services provided by the District Nursing Association or to be accommodated in the hospitals included in the Emergency Hospitals Scheme, even though they were not ill enough to go to hospital in the ordinary way."

Another outstanding feature of this war-time period was the generosity of industrial firms in offering scholarships for training in industrial nursing. Industrial nurses are grateful for their generous response and recognise this to be a tribute to the work of nurses generally in industry.

The following extracts from the Industrial Health Section of the Annual Report of the Chief Inspector of Factories give an official review of this specialised branch of nursing at this period:

Industrial Health Section in Annual Report of the Chief Inspector of Factories, 1942, by E. R. A. Merewether, M.D., M.R.C.P., F.R.S.E., Barrister-at-Law.

At the outbreak of this war there were a small number of whole-time Industrial Medical Officers, who had already formed a scientific society of their own for the study of industrial health, some 1,700 Examining Surgeons—some of whom, like Arlidge and Dearden, had long since done classical work on aspects of Industrial Health—who were carrying on valuable, if limited, preventive work in factories, and a small section of general practitioners who had specially interested themselves locally in these matters, all of whom were engaged on preventive work part or whole-time in individual factories.

A patchwork and unobtrusive service, it is true, but normal in the evolutionary stage of a British institution.

The evolution of industrial nursing was, of course, a natural corollary, and proceeded in sympathy and on parallel lines.

These services had proved their value before the outbreak of war to those employers and workers who had direct experience, but their work was little known outside these circles.

War requirements necessitated the provision of these health measures over a much wider area and power was obtained to require this by means of the Factories (Medical and Welfare Services) Order, 1940—which empowered the Chief Inspector to direct the provision of medical, nursing and welfare services in essential works. The expansion in this connection was considerable, but is now limited by the shortage of doctors and nurses. The success of this venture, although many medical and nursing recruits were ignorant of industrial health matters, is remarkable, and the supply of doctors and nurses for industry does not meet the demand. No direction to appoint a doctor or nurse has in fact been given under the above-mentioned Order; the results achieved were themselves sufficient to recommend the services from factory to factory. In fact, the industrial health services, partial in operation as they are still, fill a gap in the health services of the country which it is inconceivable can be allowed to disappear when the immediate emergencies are past.

Initiation of the doctors and nurses in their special duties in Industry was got over to an extent by short courses in Medical Schools of Universities and other teaching institutions for both doctors and nurses, and particularly for the latter by courses subsidised by the Ministry of Labour and National Service and conducted by the Royal College of Nursing. The Factory Department also issued a short Memorandum (Factory Form 327) on Medical Supervision in Factories, and the Medical Inspectors assisted individual works doctors and nurses so far as possible with guidance on the general principles.

This again was an emergency arrangement dictated by pressing necessity, and many doctors found themselves in difficulty owing to a misconception of the scope of their work.

As I have said, the work of the Industrial Medical Officer fills a gap in the health services of the country, because it is primarily concerned with the study of work and the work environment and their effects on the individual workers in his factory, and the application of such preventive and first-aid measures as are appropriate.

This is a speciality in itself, and it does not concern itself with the departures from health of the individual worker which are not related to his work or his working environment. Nor should the Works Medical Officer concern himself with advice and treatment of such ailments; in fact it is his positive duty to refer back to the private doctor all such matters, so that the worker may immediately be in a position to be advised as to appropriate treatment, and to be able to take advantage of the whole range of specialist and local authorities' medical services which are available through the worker's own doctor.

Thus there is still misconception on the function of the Industrial Medical Officer, not so much by them, as by the general public and by doctors who have not as yet interested themselves in this work.

An exact appreciation of the scope of the doctor specialising in industrial medicine is of fundamental importance if the benefits of this specialised branch of preventive medicine are to be available for all factories, small or large. As I see it, therefore, the industrial medical officer should be as much as possible about the works and as little as possible in his factory ambulance room or surgery.

Co-operation between the industrial medical officer, the private practitioner and the local health services should be complete and not a one way traffic. This is all the more important because it seems probable that the only way of catering efficiently for the industrial health needs of the great number of smaller factories is through the part-time services of general practitioners who are interested in this work and have definite special knowledge of it or will obtain it.

Too much praise cannot be given to the nurse in industry, and in this tribute I include the work of the St. John Ambulance Association, the St. Andrew's Association, and the British Red Cross Society. The number of State-registered nurses in industry continues to increase; they brought the broad outlook of special training to special industrial problems, to the additional advantage of the well-being of the worker. The fact that the State-registered nurses and the trained members of the voluntary association have different types of training does not prevent the employment of both in the same factory. As it happens, however, their work is complementary, and both have their special contribution to make.

At the end of 1942 there were approximately 850 Works Medical Officers in industry, just under 19 per cent being whole-time, and approximately 7 per cent were women. At the same time, there were roughly 4,000 hospital trained nurses; this figure has now risen to about 6,000 of whom well over 63 per cent are State-registered.

I cannot leave the subject of Medical Supervision without referring to the medical service of the Ministry of Supply. The Ministry of Supply is the largest direct employer of labour in the country in connection with the Royal Ordnance Factories which it controls. The majority of these are new factories set up for the purposes of this war often in isolated places, to which workers had to be transferred in large numbers.

A further extract from the Annual Report of the Chief Inspector of Factories for the Year 1944 reads as follows:

Medical Supervision

At the end of 1944 there were approximately 180 doctors exercising full-time medical supervision in 275 factories, and at least 890 exercising substantial medical supervision in 1,320 factories on a regular part-time basis. Since then the lesser demands of war and the commencing change-over of industry to peace-time operation have on the one hand been accompanied by a reduction in these numbers owing to closure of factories, and on the other hand have enabled some factories formerly unable to get medical and nursing personnel to install these services.

The number of women nurses in industry from the most recent figures available would seem to be about 7,600, a slight reduction on the 1943 figures. In addition there are about 200 male nurses. Some 50 per cent of the women and 10 per cent of the male nurses are State-registered.

The reduction in industrial nurses is due to the pressing needs in other nursing fields and again the Nursing Division of this Ministry with the National Advisory Council on Nurses and Midwives has done invaluable work in reconciling competitive claims on the services of nurses. A number of factory nurses volunteered with the consent of their employers to leave industry temporarily to help with battle casualties after D-day. Fortunately the extent of these casualties was so much less than had been anticipated that only a few of the volunteers from industry were called upon.

To meet the needs of industry for State-registered nurses with industrial training, the short intensive courses of instruction sponsored by the Ministry for suitable candidates over the age of 27 years have been continued.

Royal Ordnance Factories

The Medical and Nursing Services in the Royal Ordnance Factories and other establishments of the Ministry of Supply were further developed during the year. A number of medical and nursing post-graduate courses were held throughout the year and particular attention was paid to teaching the principles and practice of industrial medicine and the development of a high standard of surgical technique.

At no time has it been possible to classify industrial nursing personnel entirely according to qualifications and in each

survey made by the Chief Inspector of Factories it was estimated that a considerable percentage of the total number of
nurses employed in factories were not State-registered. That
there is a place for the State-enrolled Assistant Nurse is unques-
tioned, though adequate supervision is necessary. Dilution in
industrial as in all other branches of nursing is accepted in
principle though it seems reasonable to ask that the extent of
this dilution should be regulated by the profession itself. The
National Association of State-enrolled Assistant Nurses has
made recommendations as to a salary scale for nurses working
in industry.

One of the encouraging signs at this time was the willingness of organisations to recognise that the industrial nurse,
because of her close contact with the workers, had a contribution to give to the many social problems which developed
during the war. The British Social Hygiene Council and the
Central Council for Health Education sought her opinion on
methods of health teaching in factories and, in its widest
sense, health education is now acknowledged to be a nursing
function.

Encouraging also was a request from the Industrial Medical
Services Sub-Committee of the British Medical Association
for the Industrial Nurses' Sub-Committee of the Royal
College of Nursing to work with them in a memorandum on
the place of industrial medicine in a comprehensive health
service. Discussion with the Association of Industrial Medical
Officers was also appreciated and conferences with them
clarified some of the professional points which arose in the
rapid development of this new service.

The Council of the Royal College of Nursing set up in
1944 an Advisory Board on Nursing Education under the
Chairmanship of Sir Cyril Norwood, M.A. Its terms of
reference were: " to advise and assist the Council in imple-
menting the terms of the Royal Charter of the College in the
further promotion of nursing education and educational

policy and the institution of post-certificate educational qualifications." Consideration of the special field of industrial nursing was delegated to an Industrial Nursing Board of Studies in 1947 on which the industrial nurse was represented through the Public Health Section of the Royal College. The Universities of Birmingham, Manchester and Glasgow are also represented on the Board of Studies and joint consultation through these channels has established a valuable link between those educational bodies which are considering plans for the future educational standards and qualifications of the industrial nurse.

The growing need up and down the country prompted the Royal College of Nursing to appoint an Industrial Nursing Organiser and Miss Carol Mann, S.R.N., took up her duties in 1945. Among her wide range of responsibilities she encouraged the formation of Industrial Nurses' Discussion Groups which function within the framework of the Public Health Section of the Royal College, In addition the arranging of conferences in co-operation with industry, which continues to give generous hospitality for these popular events, has met with much success, and progress is steadily being made. The Industrial Nurses' Sub-Committee of the Public Health Section dealt with a wide variety of problems peculiar to the industrial nurse and her employer and advised the Council on the formation of College policy in this field. This Committee is representative of the country as a whole and through its powers of co-option has the advantage of the experience of nurses from a wide group of industries.

The need to organise other workers in the field of industrial health led to the formation of the Industrial Nursing Association in January 1947 with headquarters at Birmingham. Membership is open to State-registered nurses, assistant nurses and first-aid workers. One of the objects is to promote greater unity among industrial nurses and persons engaged in industrial nursing and welfare and the co-ordination of all branches of medical, nursing and industrial social service. It seeks to provide an efficient and progressive health service and to further the education of industrial nursing personnel.

During the war a National Advisory Council on the Recruitment and Distribution of Nurses and Midwives had kept the nurse-power situation continually under review and acted in an advisory capacity to the Nursing Services Branch of the Ministry of Labour. In 1943 it was renamed the National Advisory Council of Nurses and Midwives and extended its advisory function to the Ministry of Health. As D-day approached and the preparations to receive Service casualties gathered momentum, there was an official appeal to industrial nurses to return to the hospitals in readiness for the invasion and to care for battle casualties. There was an immediate response, some nurses volunteering for three months or more, their employers willingly giving them leave of absence for this purpose. During this crisis the Nursing Department of Ministry of Labour and National Service, of which Mrs. B. Bennett, O.B.E., S.R.N., D.N., was Chief Nursing Officer, carefully scrutinised all the new appointments of nurses to industry, among other circumstances home commitments and immobility being taken into consideration. Each case was judged on its own merits and a principle was established, and remains unaltered today, that industrial nursing is a suitable field for the older nurse with home ties. It is equally suitable for part-time nurses, a fact which has been clearly demonstrated in practice.

It would be wellnigh impossible for the rapid growth of industrial nursing not to encounter some opposition from many differing points of view. From an entirely unexpected quarter arguments were advanced by certain sections of the medical profession that conditions of service being asked for by the Royal College of Nursing were too favourable to the nurse and would not be accepted in industry. Furthermore, nurses were being settled in industry without medical supervision and this, too, caused some disapproval from the medical profession. It was said that the modern concept of industrial nursing was trespassing on the preserves of " Welfare " and personnel management, and efforts were made to relegate the nurse once more to the four walls of the ambulance room from which she had been struggling for release. But the industrial nurse had established the principle in her profession that she was a member of the public health nursing team and resisted all efforts to isolate her service from that of the team since they could only lead to a restriction of her influence.

Slowly but surely the opposition weakened and the wartime struggle abated.

9

Industrial Nursing and the National Health Service

A GLIMPSE OF THE FUTURE

IN the first White Paper issued in 1944 by the Minister of Health, Rt. Hon. H. V. Willink, K.C., M.P., on a National Health Service, it was stated, "The aim of the new National Health Service will be to provide every person or better still every family with a personal or family practitioner who will be able to become familiar with the circumstances of those in his care—in the home *and at work*." This statement indicated therefore that an Industrial Health Service was contemplated and would be an integral part of the proposed comprehensive Health Service. Consequently the Public Health Section of the Royal College of Nursing presented a memorandum to the Minister of Labour and National Service on the place of Industrial Nursing in the future in view of the suggested legislation. In introducing the subject it was said, "There can be no doubt that to enable a unified Industrial Health Service to be developed the ultimate authority should be the Minister of Health, though there are precedents for the delegation of certain powers to other authorities when circumstances make this desirable. In this case it seems logical to suggest that in view of existing arrangements which have stood the test of war, certain responsibilities in relation to the health of the workers should continue to be delegated to the

Ministry of Labour and National Service and that further delegation of powers to other Ministries might be desirable." The Memorandum continues, ' Whatever the final plan for linking together the existing fragmentary Health Services, it would be advisable if individual employers, when setting up Industrial Health services, took into consideration the needs of neighbouring factories in adjoining areas. The best use of nursing staff must be a ruling factor in any plans which are made." It goes on to say, " The establishment of a Central Health Service Council to advise the Minister of Health is welcomed by the Nursing profession and it is suggested that adequate representation should be given to industrial nurses on the Nursing and Midwifery section of this Council. Furthermore, it is recommended that at all organisation levels—national regional and local—adequate industrial nursing representation should be given on all advisory committees." The Memorandum then continues, " The help of the Medical Inspectors and Factory Inspectors has been greatly appreciated by nurses working in industry and much of the high standard already achieved has been due to the stimulus and encouragement given by the Factory Inspectorate generally. Industrial nurses, however, feel that if their service is to develop side by side with the Public Health Services, the nurses themselves should take a more definite part in its administration. The rapid development of the service since the war has naturally produced varying standards. Professional guidance and help for employers who are establishing an Industrial Health Service is needed. For this purpose it is suggested there should be appointed to the Factory Department of the Ministry of Labour and National Service a Chief Industrial Nursing Officer with the necessary nursing supervisory staff to assist her. Their function would be to give consultation service to employers and others in co-operation with the factory inspectorate on the initial planning and other practical details of the operation of the Service. Errors in layout or equipment, which the nurse so often finds on taking up her employment, could be obviated if professional advice were available beforehand." The need for supervision in the Industrial Nursing Service in common with all other public health services was stressed. The memorandum further emphasised fundamental principles such as the need for more facilities for improved post-certificate training, standardised conditions of service, and the employment of male nurses and anciliary nursing grades in the industrial health service under the supervision of a State-registered nurse.

The Royal College of Nursing was not entirely successful in all its recommendations at that time but recent events such as the nationalisation of the coal industry, electricity and transport, suggest that the higher administrative nursing posts will be held by industrial nurses in the future, and the position is developing satisfactorily. Mary Gardner, in *Public Health Nursing* (Journal of the National Organisation for Public Health Nurses, Inc., U.S.A.), ably expressed the need for nursing supervision when she wrote " . . . the industrial nurse, like any other nurse working alone, needs to bear constantly in mind the danger of deterioration in all unsupervised effort, and must set herself resolutely to combat this tendency by continually measuring her work by the standard of that of other women of her own profession. Without the double stimulus of approbation and criticism that is a part of all supervision, it is difficult to avoid, on the one hand, undue discouragement and, on the other, that easy satisfaction with partial accomplishment that is death to better things. . . . Real and lasting success can be attained only by the nurse who also conforms to the highest standards of her own profession."

The appointment of Chief Nursing Officers in certain industrial firms has been welcomed by the industrial nurses themselves. From isolated units having little or no contact with other community services or even the nursing profession itself, comprehensive industrial nursing services are being developed and the staff, in many cases led by a Chief Nursing Officer and other supervisory officers, assisting her are building an *esprit de corps* and pride in work which is possible in large and co-ordinated concerns.

As the Nurses' Salaries Committee (Rushcliffe) had not included the industrial nurse in its scope, the seriousness of this omission was stressed on the Memorandum sent to the Ministry of Labour and National Service and it was recommended that she should be included as soon as possible.

Much has happened since the Memorandum was presented and a comprehensive health service is now available to everyone under the provisions of the National Insurance Act, the National Health Service Act, and the National Insurance (Industrial Injuries) Act. The Industrial Health Service, however, is still largely accepted as a responsibility by industry according to the enlightment of individual employers. Furthermore, the new Whitley machinery under the National Health Service, embracing all public health nurses engaged in the service, does not at present consider the question of industrial nursing salaries and conditions of service. There is no doubt, however, that in the past the Rushcliffe salary scales have influenced, and more recently Whitley awards are influencing, salaries in industry but nursing has far to go before a fully comparable standard of service conditions exists among the various branches of the profession.

The successful functioning of the new National Health Service will always depend on the closest co-ordination of the work between industry and the National Health Services and there are indications that the industrial nurse is giving her special contribution in common with her colleagues in other fields. She often represents her management, or alternatively her profession, on advisory committees or panels which are being arranged by the Ministry of National Insurance or the Ministry of Labour and National Service and on other community groups in her neighbourhood. Such subjects as rehabilitation and resettlement of the disabled and the day-to-day administration of the new insurance legislation give wide scope for her specialised knowledge.

It is pleasure to pay tribute to the long tradition of voluntary work in the realm of first aid for the injured which has been given by St. John Ambulance Brigade and the British Red Cross Society in this country and there is no doubt that an even wider field of service is opening up before them in industry and in other spheres within the National Health Service. This is accepted generally. The Royal College of Nursing, recognising the value of discussion on the professional aspect of the work, the need for supervision of ancilliary grades, their relationship to one another and their scope and training for the work, established a Standing Conference in 1945. Representatives from the British Medical Association, the Association of Industrial Medical Officers, the St. John Ambulance Brigade and the British Red Cross Society, together with the Chief Medical Officers from certain Government Departments which are concerned, meet with the Royal College of Nursing periodically in order to formulate a joint policy on these matters.

It is a truism to say that social medicine is a changing dynamic force permeating all levels of human endeavour, and the need for continual review of the situation is obvious. With this in view the Government decided to make a critical survey of the industrial health service with particular reference to its relationship with the National Health Service. Therefore, in June 1949, the Prime Minister appointed a Committee under the Chairmanship of Judge Dale to advise on the co-ordination of the Industrial Health Service with the National Health Service. The terms of reference of the Committee were:

To examine the relationship, including any possibility of overlapping, between the preventive and curative health services provided for the population and the industrial health services, which make a call on medical man-power (doctors, nurses and auxiliary medical personnel);

To consider what measure should be taken by the Government and the other parties concerned to ensure that such medical man-power is used to the best advantage; and to make recommendations.

The members of the Committee were:

Mr. John T. Byrne, Electrical Trades Union; Dr. T. A. Lloyd Davies, Chief Medical Officer, Boots Pure Drug Co., Mr. R. R. Hyde, Director, Industrial Welfare Society; Dr. Walter Jope; Mr. K. I. Julian, Chairman South-East Metropolitan Hospital Board; Dame Anne Loughlin, former chairman of the T.U.C.; Mr. J. H. Pheazey, Standard Telephones Ltd; Dr. L. Roberts, M.O.H., Sheffield; Dr. A. T. Rogers and Sir Geoffrey Vickers, V.C., National Coal Board.

Mr. F. W. Beek, Ministry of Health, and Mr. C. H. Sissons, Ministry of Labour, were joint secretaries.

Judge Dale had been County Court Judge at Bloomsbury and Aylesbury since 1947. He was Judge at Birmingham County Court from 1937 to 1946, and at Lambeth 1946-7. In 1947 he was chairman of a committee set up by the Ministry of National Insurance to review the policy adopted in scheduling industrial diseases under the Workmen's Compensation Acts, and to advise on the selection of diseases for insurance under the National Insurance (Industrial Injuries) Act.

The absence of an industrial nurse on the Committee was challenged by the Royal College of Nursing and after considerable negotiation the Prime Minister, in answer to a question asked in the House by Viscountess Davidson (Cons. Hemel Hempstead) said he had appointed Miss H. M. Edwards, M.V.O., S.R.N., Director of Nursing Services, King Edward's Hospital Fund for London, and Miss E. M. Gosling, S.R.N., Industrial Nursing Certificate, Principal Nursing Officer, Lever Brothers and Unilever Ltd., to be members of the Committee on Industrial Health Services.

The setting up of the Dale Committee was timely. When it began its deliberations its duty was to survey, among other things, a field where thousands of industrial nurses had played a full and important part in helping to maintain industrial health during the strenuous war years. At the end of hostilities, with the consequent closing of munition works, a certain number of nurses retired from active work as a natural result. There were, however, left some thousands who were anxious to make industrial nursing their permanent field of nursing service. At the time of the survey it was thought there were 2,600 State-registered nurses and 1,400 other nursing staff employed in factories. Feelings of anxiety among this group developed, as some criticism was being voiced that numbers were working outside the hospital wards where they might more usefully be employed nursing the sick. Owing to the expansion of the National Health Service a shortage of nursing personnel was developing rapidly and the needs of the sick and the demands of hospitals and local health services raised many questions in the minds of the profession and the public generally.

In November 1950 the Report of the Committee of Enquiry on Industrial Health Services (Dale Report. Cmd. 8170) was published. It was a matter for much satisfaction to industry and to the medical and nursing professions that a recommendation was made (pending any other action which might be taken later) to lift the ban imposed on substantial further development of industrial health services. The Government accepted this recommendation at once.

The report stressed that from evidence received it had been established without doubt that there was an important place in industry for the State-registered nurse, the State-enrolled assistant nurse, and the first-aid worker. A recommendation that every effort should be made to use the services of the nurse on nursing duties and not on work which could be done adequately under her supervision by the State-enrolled assistant nurse and other first-aid workers, might at first sight appear unnecessary, though the Report wisely stressed this point which is so often overlooked.

Practical suggestions for giving adequate help for record keeping and for making fuller use of part-time nursing and auxilliary help were made.

The Report stated that existing industrial health service were most important to industry; they were in many ways complementary to the National Health Service, and should be main tained and encouraged to expand with due regard to the demands of all other health services for medical and nursing manpower. It emphasised that, for the development of a comprehensive Health Service, all existing services, both State and voluntary, must be co-ordinated. Furthermore, the voluntary provision of industrial health services by employers individually and collectively should be encouraged, though the needs of the smaller factories, unable to provide for themselves unaided, must be borne in mind.

The findings of a Committee of Enquiry on the Health Welfare and Safety in Non-Industrial Employment (Cmd. 7664) published in March 1949 (under the Chairmanship of Sir Ernest Arthur Gowers, G.B.E., K.C.B.) had previously covered the whole field of employment outside industry. This included shops, offices, hotels, restaurants and the catering industry, indoor and outdoor entertainment, agriculture, the theatre, fishing and shipping, and domestic work, etc. Taking agriculture as an example, the introduction of mechanised farm implements, the more general use of insecticides and chemical sprays, each bringing with it new hazards, emphasise the need for legislation to cover the many fields of employment where few, if any, health and safety facilities exist. In many spheres of work, other than industry, welfare services are still of meagre proportions. Bearing this in mind the Dale Committee commented that it was desirable there should eventually be some comprehensive provision for occupational health covering not only industrial establishments of all kinds, both large and small, but also the non-industrial occupations surveyed in the Gowers Report. This, however, is a long-term policy which cannot be made effective without more experience and can be implemented only after much research and experiment.

To the nursing profession generally a comment in the report brought satisfaction—" We should like to draw attention to the value of the nurse in raising and maintaining the morale of the workers in the establishment in which she is employed; we regard it as an important aspect of the employment of nurses in industry."

Finally the Dale report discussed the need for surveys and research to determine more exactly the further requirements of industry in the matter of industrial health services. Such surveys would be necessary before any plan for a national scheme for the development of industrial health services could be made. More experiments for providing medical supervision by grouping small factories would play a useful part in helping to shape the future structure. Existing group schemes in Slough, Bridgend, and Hillington, Glasgow, might well prove the value of co-operation for the well-being of the whole area.

A more definite lead to the future of " First Aid " would have strengthened the common-sense approach brought to bear on this problem by the Committee. It is recognised that the contribution of the first-aider is complementary to that of the doctor and nurse though under present conditions the absence of any clear-cut national policy detracts from the general usefulness of this grade of personnel in industry. This is owing to the lack of any uniformity in training and practice. The Dale Committee rightly stressed the need that everyone undertaking first aid treatment should be trained and recognised the existing certificates now available. Furthermore, and this is even more important, it pointed out the need for maintaining the first-aider's efficiency by continual training and wider experience. A suggestion was made that more use could be made in industrial establishments of the people being trained in first aid for Civil Defence purposes, though this could only be considered a short-term policy. The Report also suggested that it might be found practicable to extend the Factories Act requirement about training in first aid to factories employing less than 50 workers. It appears that a new title is needed for first aiders working in ambulance rooms as distinct from those who merely hold a certificate. There is need for much thought and planning between all concerned to consider this. As a natural sequence the more comprehensive training which would be given would prepare them for additional responsibilities.

The Report emphasised the fundamental principle which should underly any expansion of the use of the first aiders, that their services should be under medical or nursing supervision.

Clearly the Dale Committee were limited by their terms of reference and consequently could only pronounce on the present situation. However, a first step has been taken, useful facts have been discovered, considerable evidence has been sifted and the magnitude of the problem brought to light. It remains now for the second step to be taken but this can only be done after wide discussion and research in which the industrial nurse must play her part.

10

Later Developments

Nursing Service — (a) In the Mines.
                             (b) In the Civil Service.
                             (c) In Air Transport.
                             (d) In Transport.
                             (e) On British Railways.
                             (f) In the Hopfields and among the Fisher Girls.
                             (g) In the Post Office.
                             (h) Under the British Electricity Authority.
                             (i) Through the Dock Labour Board.
                             (j) Through Group Health Services.

(a) Nursing Service in the Mines.

The need for a nursing service in the mines had long been recognised by the Royal College of Nursing. As a step towards bringing such a service into being the College made a survey of existing health facilities in several mining districts and a memorandum based upon the information obtained in this survey was presented to the Ministry of Fuel and Power in 1943; the main recommendations were:

(a) that State-registered Nurses with industrial training should be appointed to serve at collieries.

(b) that a Nursing Advisory Service should be established within the Ministry to work in collaboration with the Ministry's medical officers.

These recommendations were accepted in principle but were not implemented at that time because of war-time conditions and, later, the plans for nationalisation of the industry.

Even so, a start was made in 1945 when the Ministry announced a policy of providing specially designed " Medical Treatment Centres " at all new pithead baths. These centres were to be staffed by state-registered nurses, assisted by the full-time and part-time first-aid attendants of whom there were large numbers already working in the first-aid rooms which the law demands shall be the minimum provision at every pit.

With the advent of the Coal Industry Nationalisation Act, 1946, all the collieries in the country, except certain very small ones, were taken over by the newly constituted National Coal Board on January 1, 1947. Such medical facilities as already existed in the industry were taken over at the same time and the services of the few State-registered nurses employed at collieries were retained. Before long the National Coal Board pronounced in favour of the policy on which the Ministry of Fuel and Power had made a start two years before. Plans were drawn up for the building of over two hundred colliery medical centres, to be located at the larger pits; generally, this meant where 700 or more men were employed. All these centres were to be staffed by State-registered nurses working under the Board's own medical staff.

Responsibility to the Board for control of the National Coal Board Medical Service was in the hands of the Chief Medical Officer at the Headquarters in London and of Divisional Medical Officers in eight of the industry's nine Divisions. The South Eastern Division, comprising only four pits, was under the general supervision of the Chief Medical Officer.

When the National Coal Board took over there were 23 State-registered nurses employed in the industry and this number had increased to 55 by the end of 1948. They were not evenly spread throughout the coalfields, for more than half were working in only two divisions. During 1948 the attendances for treatment at nurse staffed centres were 227,000, a vast increase over the attendances at the statutory first-aid rooms which preceded the new centres. This seemed to indicate that the provision of properly designed buildings and skilled staff increased the men's confidence in the service available to them and uncovered a previously hidden demand for treatment of minor injuries and sickness. It is also reasonable to assume that the pressure upon local general practitioners and out-patient departments was much decreased and a considerable saving made in productive working time.

A most important contribution is made to the work of the medical and nursing service in the mines by the trained first-aiders of the industry who have behind them a long tradition of devoted service. This, and the peculiar conditions obtaining in the pits, was recognised by the Home Office when in 1945, following representations made to them by the Ministry of Fuel and Power, permission was granted for first-aiders " employed in or about collieries " to administer morphine to injured colleagues. These men were selected and trained by doctors in the technique of giving injections. This scheme has done much to alleviate the suffering of men hurt in underground accidents, sometimes miles from the shaft bottom.

The accident rate in mining—there are about 2,000 serious accidents every year—presents many problems and not least among them is the need for rehabilitation facilities which will enabled skilled miners to regain their working capacity when it is possible to fit them for return to their original jobs in the mines. The Miners' Welfare Commission, set up in 1920 to administer the money obtained from a levy on each ton of coal raised, has done valuable work in this field. In 1948 eight rehabilitation centres, devoted exclusively to the care of injured miners, were in operation. The Commission also provided convalescent homes and more financial assistance to hospital and district nursing associations in mining areas, and provided ambulance cars. It has also sponsored research into miner's nystagmus and rheumatism.

(b) *Nursing Service in the Civil Service.*

The evacuation of large numbers of Civil Servants during the war and the present policy of the Government to maintain a system of dispersal may, perhaps, have hastened the establishment of a Medical Service for the Civil Service. Evacuation and dispersal brought social and health problems in their train, not the least being the housing of staff and their care during illness and those requiring both hospitalisation or home nursing in the temporary lodgings provided for them. The health supervision of the Civil Service, employing nearly three quarters of a million persons, presents unusual difficulties and as an example the creation of a new headquarters for the Ministry of National Insurance in Newcastle upon Tyne, where 7,000 employees are housed in one building, points, in some measure, to the future pattern of the permanent policy to be followed. Large numbers of employees in Manchester, Birmingham and other large cities emphasise the difficulties of administering a service so far away from the centre.

The appointment of Dr. W. E. Chiesman, M.D., F.R.C.P., as Chief Medical Advisor to the Treasury was the first step taken and the existing Post Office Medical Service was later incorporated in the new organisation. The policy of the Government is to employ first aiders who hold a certificate of efficiency from the British Red Cross Society or St. John Ambulance Brigade as a general rule, and nurses in establishments which are large enough or can be grouped together to make such an appointment advisable. There are facilities for looking after emergencies and in most buildings where 1,000 or more civil servants are employed a sick-room is provided and this is in the charge of a State-registered nurse. First aiders are trained in working hours and are in suitable cases assigned to the offices where fewer people are employed. Offices in Whitehall are grouped in such a way that a service of this kind is available for all. Careful consideration has been given to the scope and function of the nursing staff and because of the problems of housing and the many social disturbances which these produce there has developed a close co-operation between nurses and welfare officers in the various Government departments who are responsible for the conduct of the sick-room service.

Standing Orders in relation to treatment and the first aid of minor injuries and disorders are issued for nurses and their assistants and are endorsed by the Chief Medical Officer. This is an important point when medical supervision is sometimes remote.

(c) *Nursing Service in Air Transport.*

The nursing services now operating in the British Overseas Airways Corporation were started from small beginnings in 1938 through the inspiration of Colonel Frederick P. Mackie, ex-I.M.S., the company then being known as Imperial Airways Ltd. The Board soon realised the need for the medical side to be complemented by nursing staff and Sir John Reith decided to appoint a Matron to co-ordinate the service. The arrival of Mrs. Attwood, S.R.N., so well known in flying circles, was welcomed. As the widow of Captain E. H. Attwood, a pioneer R.F.C. and civil pilot who will long be remembered as one who blazed the trail of flying and plotted many of the air routes throughout the Empire, she was experienced in air travel and familiar with the requirements of those engaged in it. Her intimate experience of the special needs of pilots and other staff often living far from home and in unusual surroundings of Eastern cities was valuable, and a sound foundation was laid on which the Service has grown.

She remembers with amusement the office girl and the vast array of bottles which she took over from the existing first-aid service at Airways Terminal, Victoria, S.W.1, and also of the close check on her own expenditure on drugs and equipment which was kept in those early days. A sum of £5 was considered rather much for a Matron to need for petty cash!

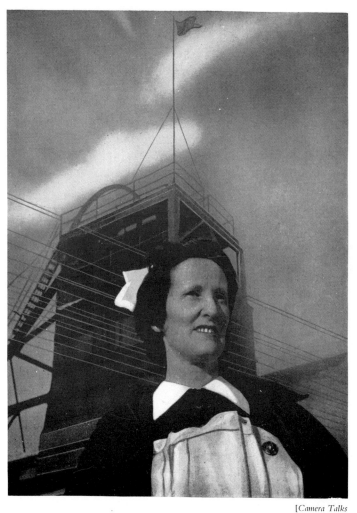

NURSING IN THE MINES

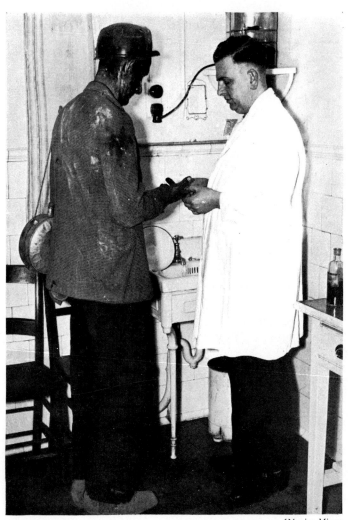

[*Nursing Mirror*

A STUDY IN BLACK AND WHITE

Cairo, Baghdad, Delhi, Karachi, Calcutta and Shannon were familiar names in her day-to-day administration and by degrees some of these bases were manned by nursing sisters, though recent changes in organisation have centralised the service in Great Britain.

Early in the last war the Company was evacuated to Bristol and Industrial Nursing Sisters, some holding the Industrial Nursing Certificates, were appointed to new depots, factories and bases as they were established, at Whitchurch, Hurn, Aldermaston, Bovingdon, Brislington, Treforest and Bath, and also at Brentford, Croydon and Filton.

The nursing duties cover Passenger Welfare, Industrial and Clinical Medicine under the supervision and co-operation of a Medical Officer at each base. The nurses are required to be State-registered, hold a certificate of the Central Midwives Board and preferably also a certificate of Industrial Training.

Each base has its Medical Department with a Nursing Sister in attendance for day-to-day first aid, supervision of hygiene and general welfare. A 24-hour service is maintained at the airports, where medical orderlies work in co-operation with the sisters under the supervision of a Medical Officer. The work covers the immunisation of all air crews, disinsectisation of planes, the collecting of drinking water specimens from the planes for bacteriological testing, and maintenance and checking of all first aid equipment as it is supplied to the different aircraft. The Department supervises the carrying out of all health regulations as laid down in the Factories Act covering heating, lighting, ventilation and sanitation.

All aircrews are required to report at periodic intervals for a medical examination, and at any time of day or night, on disembarking from overseas, they must report any illness incurred overseas or suffered in transit. Sick passengers are met on landing or embarking by the Nursing Sisters and assistance and treatment given as required. Frequently, they work in co-operation with the Port Health Officers.

Passenger Welfare includes an Immunisation Centre where passengers receive inoculations for travel to all parts of the world and here the Sister helps the doctors to smooth out many of the difficulties that arise over the required certificates and many explanations have to be given for the necessity of the inoculations. Some of these experiences prove exceedingly amusing and at other times, in emergencies, often very sad.

In addition to the general medical facilities, a Central Clinic is maintained in London for the medical examination of staff wives, children and aircrews returning from and going overseas, also the medical examinations of all new staff entering the Corporation's service.

(d) Nursing Service in Transport.

The nationalisation of transport was signalised by the setting up of a British Transport Commission, within the framework of which functional organisations operate in the special fields. These are 1. Docks and Inland Waterways Executive, 2. London Transport Executive, 3. Railways Executive, 4. Road Transport Executive, and 5. Hotels Executive.

1. A Health Service for Inland Waterways.

The life of a canal boatman is hard. There are, for instance, 96 locks to be negotiated between Birmingham and London, and the heavy winches require strong muscles to open the lock doors. A brave heart only can endure the life. In the early days the boats were all horse drawn. The life was healthy, for the boatman and his family walked miles on the tow-path and exercise was good as a contrast to the cramped living conditions on the boat, but by degrees motor power was substituted. The picturesque canal boats, in which the boatmen take so much pride, are a familiar sight on the waterways meandering through the Midlands and near London, though the origin of the traditional design is sunk in oblivion. The medieval castle, wreaths of red and pink roses, and hearts are motifs which occur with regularity in the design on the spick and span painted canal boats, and the shining brass water jugs, cooking utensils and tiller are equally a pride to the boatman's wife. Such a job brings dangers in its train and sudden illness, far from the centres of habitation, must be dealt with.

On the banks of the Grand Union Canal which flows through the Northamptonshire village of Stoke Bruerne, near Towcester, there had been for several generations a store where the needs of the canal boats could be met. Rope was a necessity, as all the boats were drawn by horses on the tow-paths, and at this same spot was a rope-walk where the manufacture of rope and twine was carried on. To this home, to care for her father, returned the daughter of the family, who was a nurse. Familiar with the comings and goings of the boatmen past her home and their work in negotiating one of the locks outside her front door, she found herself in the centre of a new industrial field. Practical help was first given voluntarily by this pioneer family, but later, realising the need for an organised service, the owners of the canal boats arranged for the work to be subsidised. The firms combining in the plan— later merged into the Inland Waterways—were: Grand Union Canal Carrying Company Ltd., London; Fellows, Morton and Clayton Ltd., Birmingham; Wander Bros., Ovaltine Works, King's Langley; Samuel Barlow Ltd., Tamworth; E. E. Barlow & Sons, Birmingham; and I. B. Faulkner, Leighton Buzzard.

To the well-equipped surgery on the banks of the picturesque canal come the patients, or the nurse may go on call to tend sudden illness or accident. She frequently has to summon an ambulance and take her patient to London or other hospitals for treatment. Her opportunities for health teaching are many. Before the war the canal boatmen were well fed, their diet consisting chiefly of butter, lard, dripping, eggs and fat bacon, and the frying pan was a necessary article of the cabin equipment. These are now substituted by bread and potatoes and meagre rations which are not easy for such a floating population to supplement by fresh food and milk.

The value of this service to the employer is obvious. By daily report from the nurse he knows the movements of his men and the comings and goings of his boats. The wide social implications of this occupation are well known also to the nurse and her help and advice on a variety of human needs is appreciated by the employers and canal boat people themselves.

This one solitary industrial nurse, Mrs. Mary Ward, whose work on the canals has been described, was inherited by the Docks and Inland Waterways Executive when she was handed over by the Grand Union Carrying Company. Nationalisation has had little effect on her sphere of influence except perhaps that more boats are working in the " stretch " of canal which passes her picturesque and romantic ambulance room on the banks of the Grand Union Canal at Stoke Bruerne, near Towcester.

The lack of trained captains who know the ways of canals and locks is frustrating attempts to restrict the work to men, and the long tradition of family life aboard the canal boats is not readily disturbed. Women and children are still to be seen as part of the charming picture of boat life along the network of inland waterways meandering through the countryside. It seems that an opportunity to develop a comprehensive service for this special floating population comes into the industrial nurses' horizon, though perhaps it cannot be designed along the orthodox lines which are general in other branches of industry.

It was to the Duke of Bridgewater that the inspiration to construct a network of almost 2,000 miles of canal in this country came at a time when the costs of transport by means of the new steam engines were rising. A new and almost unknown race of boatmen (how they dislike being confused with bargemen) came into being. They have a language of their own and among their picturesque fleets number " narrow boats ", " fly boats " and " joshers ", " butty boats " and " number ones ". The helmsman may be called a " peg wiggler " or " pobblehind " and a canal is always a " cut ". This romantic setting is not, however, without its social problems. The education of the children of this nomadic group is fraught with difficulties. Special boarding schools are provided near certain main canal depots, but it is feared if these are developed the mothers will want always to be near their children and as the woman is an essential part of the boatman's team any disturbance of the present method might seriously disturb the economic basis on which the canal industry is administered. Moreover, the children themselves, so essentially part of the canal life, are the best source of recruits for the industry, and after a life ashore may not regain the taste for life as a " water gipsy ". However, it seems necessary, if this industry is to develop, for the boatman to be provided with an adequate wage which will enable him to maintain a home ashore where his family, at least during the early years, may be safely housed while he is absent. This problem arising from many social maladjustments is ever present in the daily life of the one and only industrial nurse working on the canals, but the day may come when a complete service will be provided and the British Transport Commission can give attention to this charming picture of English canal life.

2. London Transport Executive.

It is over a century since George Shillibeer operated the first horse-bus in London for public hire. The Shillibeer bus ran between the Yorkshire Stingo, Marylebone Road, London, and the Bank in 1829 for a sixpenny fare. This was the beginning of London's public transport system; the London General Omnibus Company was later established in 1856, and the Metropolitan Railway in 1863. Through the successive stages of amalgamation of the Underground Group of Companies to the establishment of the London Passenger Transport Board in 1933 and of the London Transport Executive in 1948, is a story of rapid expansion and development to provide London's present-day efficient transport service. The amalgamation to form one working unit, the London Passenger Transport Board, was largely the work of one man—Albert Stanley, later Lord Ashfield. This vast organisation employs approximately 100,000 persons. There are 112 garages and depots, each employing from 300 to 1,000 men, 3 generating stations and some 280 railway stations. The industrial canteen service is one of the largest in the country, comprising 184 canteens and a number of mobile canteens. At the main repair works at Chiswick, Charlton, Acton and Aldenham, where some 10,000 people are employed, there are well-equipped works surgeries staffed by seven State-registered nurses. Many of the employees, as is natural in a transport organisation, are out on the road or railway for almost the whole of their daily work. Trained first aid men are employed at the garages and railway depots. Training of first aid men has a long and successful tradition in the transport service, which is continued by the London Transport Ambulance Centre of the St. John Ambulance Association. Classes in first aid are arranged and in accordance with the Factories Act, trained men and women are employed as first-aiders throughout the service. No full-time first-aiders are employed.

(e) *Nursing Service on British Railways.*

The Medical Service of the British Railways today represents the development of a service which existed in each Company during the War, and which was expanded then to include emergency medical services for all the railways. Thus first aid posts were established and were manned by State-registered nurses at most of the London termini and at the large provincial stations. State-registered nurses were also working in the dressing stations in many railway works, although the railway hospitals have since been taken over by the Ministry of Health.

Prior to nationalisation, the Great Western Medical Fund Hospital Scheme provided a General Hospital at Swindon with dental and other anciliary services for railwaymen, their wives and families, which was maintained by contributions from the men, augmented by a financial grant from the Railway Company. The hospital was staffed with State-registered nurses and was a very successful undertaking until the premises were acquired by the Oxford Regional Medical Board of the National Health Service. Similarly, the London, Midland and Scottish Accident Hospital, Mill Street, Crewe, provided a Hospital Service for the railway employees at Crewe, including a special Orthopaedic and Rehabilitation Centre, and was staffed by a matron and State-registered nurses. This work, developed under the guidance of Dr. H. E. Moore, O.B.E., M.B., Ch.B., was a pioneer venture and demonstrated how much could be done for disabled railway-men.

The Medical Service was reorganised and extended after nationalisation of the railways, when the Nursing Service developed, both being in charge of the Chief Medical Officer, British Railways. The Railway Medical Service also covers the requirements of the Road Haulage, Docks and Inland Waterways, and the Hotels Executives, representing 730,000 employees in all.

The Nursing Service of British Railways now provides the Nursing Staffs for the dressing stations and medical centres at works, railway termini and elsewhere, where a large number of workers are employed. This service, which offers a full-time appointment to State-registered nurses, is still expanding, although the final plan of the organisation is not yet approved.

(f) *Nursing Service in the Hopfields and among the Fisher Girls.*

An interesting and useful experiment in industrial nursing

in a seasonal industry is centred on the hopfields in Kent and has been carried on for a number of years. It was to Father Richard Wilson, a Stepney clergyman, that the desire to help the " hopping " community first came. Large numbers of his own parishioners migrated annually for the season to the district of Five Oak Green, Kent, and on one of his frequent visits to care for their spiritual welfare he found conditions which were terrible. Even the essentials of life were absent; shelter was meagre, the water supply no better than the farm-yard pond; no medical or nursing care available and old folk were allowed to die unattended. One day he met on the road a mother in great distress as she clasped her dead child wrapped in a parcel to her breast. Unhappiness marred what could have been a real holiday and the memory remained as a haunting nightmare. In 1898 Father Wilson was inspired to launch a practical experiment and a room in the village of Five Oak Green was hired for a hospital. Nurses from London went down to look after the hop-pickers. Smallpox patients were not unknown. Much of the service was given voluntarily both by the doctors and nurses. The needs of this migrant population grew rapidly and one room gave way to a small house. This in turn became too small and Father Wilson next purchased the Rose and Crown Inn in the village, which was adapted as a hospital. After his death in 1926 the present building called The Little Hoppers Hospital was set up as a memorial to his pioneering enterprise.

During the hop harvest a doctor visits the hospital twice a day and the staff is a matron, a State-registered nurse and Red Cross nursing help. There are also four dispensaries attached to the hospital situated on neighbouring farms and a State-registered nurse is in charge of the work there. Nor are the spiritual and social needs of the hoppers forgotton. Sunday Schools and Church Services are arranged and instructive film shows provided. Refreshment is taken to the fields by means of tea trolleys and canteens provide more substantial

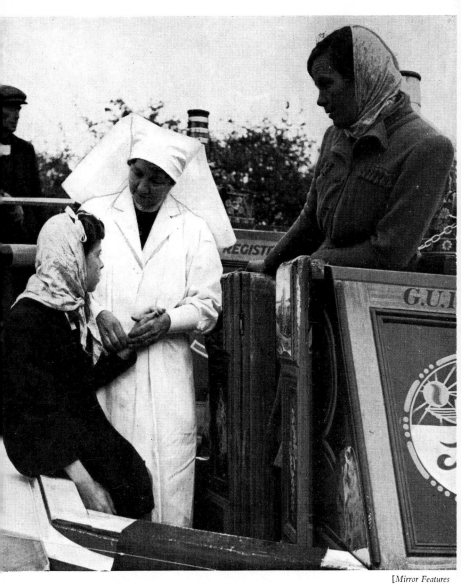

HEALTH TEACHING IN A ROMANTIC SETTING

meals. When the day is done, organised games and dancing are available for the young, and for those who like a gossip or quiet meditation a corner can be found.

In some districts the British Red Cross Society has manned this pioneer venture by hundreds of volunteers connected with their local detachments. Specially equipped dispensaries which are scattered through the hop farms now number between 30 and 40 and these are opened annually from the end of August to the end of September. A State-registered nurse is in charge of the unit and the organisation of volunteer auxiliaries to help her is a striking example of how a particular need can be met by co-operative effort.

It is not generally realised what a change is made in the life of a quiet Kentish village during the invasion of the hop-picking community, the numbers arriving from the East End of London, from Bermondsey or Southwark varying from 2,000 to 12,000 in certain areas. Whole families migrate for the hopping period which is looked forward to as an oppor-tunity for a communal holiday and is, in many instances, the only change in the year which the mother can enjoy with her family. The scene is colourful, the hop gardens are filled with women and children laughing and chattering, usually wearing gay-coloured scarves, all busy stripping the hops into the bins. The men do the heavier work of pulling down the great clusters of fruit for the stripping and moving the heavy bins when required. When the bins are filled they are taken to the oast-houses and their contents baked, and then the well-known " malty " smell comes on the air.

It is natural that calls for first aid should come along; cuts and burns, some trivial, some more serious, are the most usual injuries; hop rash has to be dealt with, and there is a careful look-out for infectious diseases and other minor ail-ments. Special cases are kept for the doctor's visit, or are taken to his surgery. There are also housing and sanitation problems to be met, but the farmers have gone far in establishing permanent hutments where the people can live in comparative comfort though picnicking is thought to be part of the fun. The Red Cross dispensaries are looked upon as centres where advice on any subject can be obtained. The staff must know when local buses depart or trains from London arrive; lost luggage must be traced and missing children are a daily anxiety. So vast a community presents still greater problems and resourcefulness and ingenuity are needed by nursing staffs who feel attracted to this particular field of activity. The well-trained public health nurse grasps the many opportunities which present themselves to her. She must be ready to deal with any emergency whether it be the harassed and distraught father who suddenly shows signs of a mental breakdown, or the baby who, finding father's bottle of beer under the hedge, drinks it with consequences of drunkenness and other unusual symptoms.

Other philanthropic agencies have concerned themselves with welfare work among the hoppers, and the Hop Pickers Mission, under the auspices of the Church of England Temperance Society, should be mentioned as another pioneer in this unique and interesting industry.

The story of Whitbreads, founded in 1742 and still standing on the original site in the Cripplegate Ward of the City of London, is long and fascinating, but a chief interest to many is the fact that in 1871 Louis Pasteur, during his investigation of the processes of fermentation in beer, worked in Whitbread's brewery. The microscope he used is still in working order and remains a symbol of his outstanding genius which, beginning with research into the diseases which attacked the vine and fermentation in wine, led to a revolution in medical practice. Another unique contribution which Whitbreads have given to the life of London is remembered when their handsome dray horses are seen in the streets. For over a hundred years two horses, harnessed in scarlet trappings, have drawn the coach of the Speaker of the House of Commons on important official occasions. The drayman and stablemen are Whitbread employees and the perfect setting into which these fine horses and those who care for them fit is a reflection of the high standard of welfare in the Whitbread stables.

At Paddock Wood the hoppers going to the Kentish hopfields owned by Whitbreads are provided with a health and welfare service by the firm. For those working on the Beltring and Stilstead farms, covering 1,100 acres in the Garden of England, local medical attention is available. The Salvation Army assist generally in social work, but apart from the daily visit of the doctor, the medical services are run on a voluntary basis by the Trinity College, Oxford, Mission with the assistance of medical students. The Franciscan Friary, Fern Abbas, also provides the help of a trained nurse who is assisted by monks who are members of the Catholic Mission.

The climax of the hopping season is the Hop Festival which is held in the first week in September. The hopfields are in gala mood for the occasion when a varied programme of events is provided for the pickers and the large numbers of visitors who go down for this special event. At such times a Shakespearian play, produced by "The Taverners", may be billed or a performance of "Much Binding in the Marsh", with original cast, arranged for the hoppers' entertainment. The Hop Queen will be crowned with due ceremony and the crowd is amused by an endless programme of competitions and other interesting events.

Another unusual example of seasonal industrial health work can be described, which is carried out under the auspices of the Church of Scotland. A special Fishing Stations Committee is responsible for administering a welfare service for the herring fishing fleet. During the summer season the fleet is fishing as far north as the Shetland Islands and as the herring shoals move southward past Aberdeen and down the Scottish coast, so the trawlers follow until in October to the end of November the work is centred in the waters around Lowestoft and Great Yarmouth

The Scots fisher girls also follow the boats and at one time as many as 1,200 may be stationed at Great Yarmouth. Here on the quayside they gut the fish and their skill and agility must be seen to be believed. The trawler fleet may number 200, each carrying a crew of nine or ten men. The Church of Scotland carries the entire financial responsibility of this work. To meet the immediate needs of this population, up-to-date floating medical clinics are also established on the quayside in easy access of the fisher girls and the crews of the boats when ashore.

This influx of industrial workers brings with it many social problems. Lodgings must be found, sick-bays established, canteens set up among the curing yards, and rest centres arranged. Welfare workers are available to look after their needs. State-registered nurses, assisted by other auxiliaries, tend those in need. The chief ailments are boils, septic sores, often caused by the salt water, gastric and chest complaints. Accidents occur on board the trawlers and burns are common. Fractures or severe bruising of ribs sometimes result from heavy work when the trawlers are at sea.

As December advances the herring fleet and the fisher girls return home to await next year's harvest of the seas.

(g) Nursing Service in the Post Office.

The development of the Post Office Medical Service has a long and interesting history dating back to 1854 when a temporary medical officer was appointed at the Head Post Office in London at a time when a cholera epidemic was raging in the metropolis. A year later, in 1855, when the majority of the post office staff, including letter carriers, became civil servants it was decided to appoint a whole-time permanent medical officer. This post was held by Dr. Waller Lewis. It was at first intended that his duties should be mainly supervisory, to prevent unnecessary sick absence and to ensure that letter carriers and others were physically and mentally capable of carrying out their duties efficiently. But it was soon agreed that this end could best be achieved if the lower ranks were given free medical treatment both at their offices and in their homes. News of the success of the service in London spread rapidly and brought requests for similiar consideration from other cities; Liverpool, Glasgow, Edinburgh and Dublin appointed doctors for this purpose and by the end of the century the service covered the whole country. This is probably one of the earliest examples in this country of a personal health service provided by the State. The fact that the method of payment of doctors was by capitation fee, which method was later taken as the model on which the first National Health Insurance Act was moulded, shows how sound were the foundations on which this early service was built. So similiar were the two schemes that post office officials whose salaries did not exceed £295 (£310 on London) were exempt from contributing under this Act and the Post Office system of medical treatment for these grades was retained until the introduction of the National Health Service Act in 1948.

In many directions the Service has done pioneer work. Medical examinations were given to new entrants and it has always been maintained by those who guided the development of the Service that the employment of 2,600 part-time local medical officers who were familiar with the actual conditions of work of those whose health they supervised was a strong recommendation for the method adopted.

Unusual problems presented themselves to the Post Office service in the early days. The danger of infection through sorting and handling letters and parcels and the attendance at the office of contacts with infectious disease at home remained over the years a matter of controversy, though the advice of leading epidemiologists, supported by experience in the Post Office, at last put an end to the tremendous waste of time which was enforced in many industries through out-of-date quarantine requirements.

A woman doctor was appointed in 1883 and it is on record that a female assistant was employed to help her with simple dressings and treatments. Such assistants were usually upgraded from the female staff and were known as Matrons. They were responsible for welfare duties and for generally keeping a motherly eye on the very large staff of young girls and women employed in Central London. Although 1883 saw the first appointment of a female assistant there is a strong suggestion that since the inception of the service women were employed to help the doctors, though no records of this can be traced.

The first use made of the State-registered nurse by the Post Office was in 1939 when the staffing of sick-bays provided for evacuated office staff became an urgent requirement. Recruitment was haphazard and sometimes erstwhile nurses who had taken Post Office appointments were drafted back into the health service. It was not, however, until 1945 that industrial nurses were employed and Miss Mary Wheatley, S.R.N., was the first State-registered nurse to be appointed to the General Post Office Headquarters Medical Branch. In a few large offices and training schools State-registered nurses are now employed, but one of the features of the Post Office is that its staff is widely spread over the country in small units which do not lend themselves readily to the employment of nursing personnel generally.

An interesting feature of this Health Service is that supervisory officers in the Post Office have always undertaken an element of responsibility with regard to the welfare of the staff. In modern industrial organisation they may be likened to welfare officers. A section of establishment known as " sickduty " dealing with sick leave, sick pay, preferential duties on sickness grounds on the advice of the Post Office Medical Officer, has been in operation since the middle of the nineteenth century. In fact a large measure of welfare work always characterised the Post Office Medical Service and a happy

co-operation between officers of the Post Office Staff Associations and the Medical Branch illustrates how much can be
done by mutual understanding and a willingness to work
together. A total pay-roll of approximately 330,000 people
indicates how wide are the ramifications of the postal system
and how intricate will be the health and welfare services, which
behind the scenes silently oil the wheels to ensure the prompt
and regular delivery of letters from the postman's bag and the
smooth working of the complex telephone and telegraph
systems.

It is perhaps in the pioneer work of health records that the
Post Office Medical Service is best known to industrial nurses.
Unfortunately the date when recording was commenced is not
now known, but the morbidity and mortality statistics
compiled since 1891 show interesting trends and the methods
used in keeping and compiling these have stood the test of
time. They serve as a guide to industry generally and have
gained a wide recognition of the value of Post Office methods
of sickness supervision and sick rates. Sick absence in relation
to hours of work; the effect of age distribution on sick rates;
male sick rates in occupational groups; female sick rates in
geographical distribution; sick rates in relation to adolescents
such as messenger boys and girl probationers; sick rates for
disabled persons, a major problem because of the large proportion of disabled ex-servicemen since the 1914-18 war, have
been carefully worked out and it is to Sir Henry Bashford,
M.D., F.R.C.P., until recently Chief Medical Officer for this
Service, that credit is due for this wide experiment in one
aspect of social medicine which was continually under review
in his department.

The Post Office Medical Service altered its name and became
the Post Office Branch of the Treasury Medical Service in
June 1948; although the treatment of patients, except for
emergencies, is no longer part of the service, its other functions
continue.

(h) *Nursing Service under the British Electricity Authority.*

Vesting Day for the electricity industry was April 1, 1948, following the passing of the Electricity Act of 1947.

Part I, Section I (1) of the Act reads:

" There shall be established an Authority to be known as the British Electricity Authority, and it shall be the duty of that authority, as and from the vesting date to develop and maintain an efficient, co-ordinated and economical system of electricity supply for all parts of Great Britain, except the North of Scotland, and for that purpose:

(a) to generate or acquire supplies of electricity,

(b) to provide bulk supplies of electricity for the Area Boards, hereinafter established for distribution by those Boards."

Furthermore, Part I, Section I (6), reads:

" In exercising and performing their functions the Electricity Boards shall promote the welfare health and safety of persons in the employment of the Boards."

It will be seen that a vast welfare organisation must be developed to meet the needs of the many thousands of employees centred in the power house, manufacturing and distributing units and the selling staffs throughout the 14 Area Boards administered by the British Electricity Authority.

A first step was taken in the appointment of Dr. P. Pringle, LL.B., M.R.C.S., L.R.C.P., D.I.H., Barrister at Law, as Chief Medical Officer. The parallel nursing appointment of Miss Helen M. Cousens, S.R.N., R.S.C.N., S.C.M., H.V.Cert., as Chief Nursing Officer was welcomed by the profession. An interesting innovation in the Medical Department is the creation of a new post, that of First Aid Organiser.

(i) *Nursing Service through the Dock Labour Board.*

The decasualising of dock labour and the formation of the National Dock Labour Board, controlling the employment of 76,000 dockers at 72 ports in the country, raised the whole question of health and welfare for a new group formerly deprived of the usual amenities of industrial employment.

The guaranteed wage for dockers offered a new charter of freedom to this vast army of men for whom little had been done previously. Formerly, welfare provisions now familiar in other industrial fields were entirely lacking on the dockside, and from nothing a new service is steadily being built. Sanitary arrangements, drinking water, protective clothing, canteens, had to be provided. The need for baths for men who handle dirty cargoes is still urgent though plans for these at the dockside are contemplated.

During the war years an outstanding development was initiated by the Ministry of War Transport by the creation of the Mersey Docks Medical Service and later a similiar service by the Clyde Navigation Trust. These were later taken over by the National Dock Labour Board. By the end of 1948 this service had been extended to docks at Glasgow, Liverpool, Bristol, Cardiff and Dundee. Other centres are being planned at Leith, Newcastle upon Tyne, Hull, Grimsby, London and Southampton. A service of 32 State-registered nurses operates between the docks where the service has already been established. A rehabilitation centre at Salford employing a physiotherapist and physical training instructor is maintained by the Board. From evidence given to the Committee of Enquiry, under the chairmanship of Sir Frederick Leggett, C.B., to study unofficial stoppages in the London docks, it was clear that an absence of " welfare " amenities in the London docks is a predisposing cause of the unrest. The meagre provision of first aid equipment, sanitary accommodation, washing facilities, supplies of drinking water, etc., called for much comment and agitation. The handling of " dirty " cargoes was also an important factor in the case.

It was only in the latter part of 1949 that the London docks were provided with their first medical centre, although some such centres had been operating for many years on some of the other ports. Evidence was given to the Committee that the medical centres had done much to raise the morale of the workers in the areas concerned. From Swansea came the report: " The medical centre on the docks has done much to promote industrial goodwill and to translate into reality in the minds of the men some of the objectives of the Dock Labour Scheme. Countless working hours have been saved which would otherwise have been lost by men attending doctors' surgeries or hospitals for treatment and in the days of manpower shortage this is a matter of national importance. The presence of a skilled nurse at an accident, pending the arrival of an ambulance, has saved more than one life during recent months." It is therefore apparent that a new era for the dock labourer is dawning and the popularity of the week-end schools for the men where topics such as Trade Unionism, the country's industrial needs and other economic subjects are discussed, points to a happy evolution of an organised body of men from the chaos so characteristic of casual labour before the war.

(j) Nursing Services through Group Health Services.

An estimate that 91 per cent of factories in Britain employ less than 100 workers always raises a point that it would be uneconomical to suggest the employment of an industrial nurse in the small unit, although it must be accepted that these workers need and should be given a service similiar to that provided by the larger firms. The question is how can it be maintained? The logical answer seems to be a grouping of factories geographically convenient to one another and a unique experiment at St. Mary Cray, Kent, under the auspicies of the Cray Valley Industrial Association Ltd., has demonstrated what can be done by mutual co-operation and goodwill among neighbouring factories. This Association, which was founded in March, 1942, by a group of nineteen industries situated within the Cray Valley area, included among its many activities the provision of a Medical Clinic, which was opened by Mr. George Tomlinson, Parliamentary Secretary to the Minister of Labour and National Service, on April 23, 1943, for the benefit of the workers of those member firms who wish to participate. The firms participating are diverse and include a modern bakery, a building contractor, metal welders, papermills, oil refineries and manufacturers of electrical appliances, rubber goods, printing inks, fibre suit-cases, etc. Once the decision had been made in 1942 to inaugurate a health service, steps were taken to approach the Ministry of Health and the local doctors for advice, approval and co-operation, all of which were obtained in full measure. In the initial stages a per capita charge of 12s. was levied from each member firm. Eleven companies with an aggregate payroll of approximately 1,400 people, subscribed to the service. No contribution was asked from the workers.

The venture was, from the beginning, entrusted to Miss M. Chatterton, S.C.M., with wide experience as a Health Visitor as well of industrial nursing in various industries. With the growth of services, it was found necessary to expand the staff to three in 1944, by the appointment of two State-registered nurses holding the Industrial Nursing Certificate. Twelve local practitioners, serving on a rota, gave service in the clinic of one hour on one afternoon a week, thus making a minimum demand on their time. The inclusion of a lady doctor on the panel appeals to the large number of women workers.

Among the services originally offered to member firms, though these have been modified from time to time, are:

1. Examination at the clinic of juveniles between the age of 15 and 18 years by appointed factory doctors.
2. Interviewing of new applicants and recording of a short case-history by the clinic nurse. This procedure has been found helpful, for example, in the prevention of industrial dermatitis through unsuitable work.
3. Sight-testing.
4. Personal hygiene supervision.
5. Treatment of accidents and industrial eye injuries, skin troubles, gastric disorders, boils and septic conditions, burns and the common cold, etc.

6. Daily visits to individual factories by the nursing staff who are cyclists. By these visits it is possible to extend prophylactic measures, particularly against colds, and to advise member firms on the correct and regular measures against eye injuries, dermatitis, etc.
7. Visits to sick and convalescent workers prove a valuable means of contact.
8. Regular weekly visits to the clinic of a qualified chiropodist for whose sessions advance appointments are booked.
9. The services of a consultant are available for serious eye injuries.
10. Immediate attendance at a factory where a serious accident has occurred.
11. Advice to managements as to the suitable employment of disabled persons.

In the first instance the function of the service was announced to workers by a leaflet distributed in their pay packets. Existing first aid workers in the factories were integrated with the scheme and lectures arranged to maintain interest and efficiency and to impart knowledge of up-to-date first aid equipment and its uses. Close co-operation between management and workpeople has been maintained and is best achieved through first aid and welfare personnel. It has been found necessary to stress continually the importance of reporting immediately all injuries which have necessitated an initial first aid treatment, and sepsis has been reduced in this way. The service maintains close co-operation with doctors, hospitals and other health workers and doctors find that their time, as well as that of their patients, can be saved where, after an initial visit to a doctor, prescribed treatment can be carried out and reported on by a nurse. Apart from staff expansion, concrete evidence of the growth of the service can be seen in the following treatment figures from its inception to the present time.

Year	Number of Firms	Attendance
1943-4	11	7,042
1944-5	9	6,798
1945-6	9	11,674
1946-7	10	15,536

Confidence and co-operation are the basis on which the service is being gradually built up.

An example of a Group Health Service covering a much wider area is a pioneer venture at Slough, Buckinghamshire. The Nuffield Health and Hospital Service, assisted by grants from the Nuffield Foundation, the Nuffield Provincial Hospitals Trust and Slough Estates Limited, has established a combined Industrial Health General Rehabilitation and Research Service there. There are 300 factories in the Slough area, employing approximately 30,000 persons and of this number 140 firms with 15,000 workers have joined this scheme. A valuable experiment is being worked out at Slough, showing how an industrial health service for a large group of small factories can be provided. The nursing staff consists of a superintendent of nursing, nine full-time State-registered nurses, two part-time State-registered nurses and one full-time first aid worker. Also under the professional supervision of the service are four State-registered nurses, eleven assistant nurses and two first aid workers, who are employed by larger firms in their own medical departments. As part of the plans to develop a complete recuperative centre, Farnham Park, a large country house near Slough, has been converted into a residence for industrial workers needing rehabilitation. It is an integral part of the Industrial Health Service and accommodation is provided for 63 in-patients and up to 20 outpatients. This home maintains close liaison with local hospital services and operates workshops where patients receive remedial exercises, physiotherapy, and educational and recreational training.

A unique feature of this organisation is a mobile clinic which, complete with doctor, nurse and chauffeur, tours the estate, parking at strategic spots during prearranged periods in the day. Patients needing treatment or medical care are able to avail themselves of this facility, so avoiding the journey to the central clinic. In this way a great saving of time is made.

It is estimated that some 2,000 man hours per month are saved to local industry by this mobile unit.

Recent developments have been the provision of an occupational hygiene team consisting of a medical officer and engineer who hold joint appointments with this service and the London School of Hygiene and Tropical Medicine, and a social service department under the supervision of a trained social worker.

It is encouraging to know that group health services are being developed on other industrial estates, notably at Hillington, Glasgow; Bridgend, Glamorgan; Enfield, Middlesex; Slaithwaite, Yorkshire; and others are contemplated. Another example of how a part-time industrial nursing service can be operated has been by joint co-operation with District Nursing Associations. For many years there have been instances where the Queen's Nurse has been employed by factories on a part-time or hourly basis. Her visits are timed for the convenience of the workers and the management pay for her services on a sessional basis. Services of this kind have worked satisfactorily in Birmingham, Bolton, Grimsby, Street, and Berkhamsted in Hertfordshire. For certain small factories such a plan has many advantages and the opportunities for following up cases of sickness in the home are readily recognised by the district nurse. Owing to the shortage of doctors and nurses, group health services of different kinds will no doubt play an important part in the future.

11

Some Other Influences

1. Rehabilitation and resettlement of the disabled.
2. Industrial Nursing Service and national economy.
3. Continued education in Industry.
4. Industrial Nursing Service develops overseas.
5. Spiritual values in Industry.

1. *Rehabilitation and resettlement of the disabled.*

THE continuation of a modified system of home work since industry has been concentrated within factory buildings has developed its own particular needs. The concentration in the homes of much of the wholesale clothing and dressmaking trade, french polishing, toymaking and stocking manufacturing, particularly in the villages of Derbyshire and Nottinghamshire, suggests that the nursing supervision of the health of these workers is one which could, in the future, rightly be shared between the district nurse and the health visitor, who are, in many circumstances, already visiting in the homes in the course of their normal duties. In this respect therefore, the home worker in this country is already provided with a comprehensive health service though one not usually considered as an occupational health service. It is, however, a service which presents wide possibilities and its integration with the factory health service must be considered in future planning.

The Statutory requirements in respect of " outworkers " are to be found in Section 48 of the Factories Act Abstract 1939 and 1948 which is as follows:

OUTWORKERS—Where work of certain kinds (specified by Regulations) is given to a workman or contractor to be done outside the factory, a list of all such persons must be kept in the prescribed form, and a copy of the list must be sent to the Local Authority during February and August in each year. The requirement applies irrespective of whether the materials for the work are supplied by the occupier or not.

This work falls within the function of the Sanitary Inspector and the supervision he exercises deals chiefly with suitability of premises where the home work is done, the detection of overcrowding and the control of infectious disease. Where action is required it is taken against the employer through the Medical Officer of Health of the Local Authority.

A disabled person has been defined as " one who, on account of injury, disease or congenital deformity, is substantially handicapped in obtaining or keeping employment, or in undertaking work on his own account of a kind which, apart from that injury, disease or deformity, would be suited to his age, experience and qualifications." Owing to the great interest now being taken in the welfare of disabled men and women, a wide field of opportunity now opens up before them, and in consequence a rapidly increasing group of " outworkers " is taking its place in industrial production. Although so many of these are " homebound " and in many cases confined to bed or a wheel chair, they are now able to become, in many instances, more or less self-supporting and, if given suitable training and facilities, can be regarded as productive workers once again. Fortunately the lot of these patients is not so unhappy as in the past.

The British Council for Rehabilitation which was established in February 1944 has done much to focus the attention of the country on the need for a deeper understanding of the position and the requirements of physically and mentally handicapped persons. Much of the credit for the inception of this idea for bringing together all the organisations interested in rehabilitation can be attributed to the inspiration and determination of the late Dame Georgiana Buller, D.B.E.,

R.R.C. She was elected as the Council's first Chairman. The main objects of the Council are:

(a) To act as a central co-ordinating body for the various interests concerned in the widest aspects of Rehabilitation.

(b) To promote and correlate courses of study in Rehabilitation in all its aspects and to provide opportunities for workers in each section to study the subject as a whole.

(c) To invite the active co-operation of Government Departments, Hospitals, Universities, Training Colleges, Educational Institutions and Research Foundations in promoting the study and practice of Rehabilitation.

(d) To secure the active co-operation and participation of Commerce, Industry and Professional Bodies in the problems of resettlement.

" Rehabilitation ", according to the Constitution of the British Council, " covers the whole range of services from the time of the onset of the individual's disability to the point at which he is restored to normal activity or the nearest possible approach to it."

From this definition it will be seen that nursing will play an important part. all through the process of recovery. The hospital team, the industrial nurse, the health visitor and district nurse, each a cog in the functional wheel, will play her respective part in this service of rehabilitation and resettlement. There is, perhaps, no other field in social medicine and nursing where a dovetailing of effort is so much needed, because of the many facets to the problems which are involved.

Consequently, since the Disabled Persons (Employment) Act, 1944, was placed upon the Statute Book, yet another field of opportunity has opened up to public health nurses who are visitors in the homes of the people and who, from their privileged position, know of many of the human tragedies which are hidden there. This perhaps refers chiefly to the district nurse and health visitor who may be visiting disabled patients. Many of these may be sheltered from the unkind blasts of the outside world by devoted and self-sacrificing parents, but could enjoy a fuller life if given the opportunity to express themselves through suitable activity. Public health nurses discover such patients in the course of their work and can call to their assistance those social agencies which can best help in planning a suitable programme for them. The nurses must, however, first recognise the need and take suitable steps to meet it.

The provision of educational and preparatory training facilities for long stay patients in hospitals and sanatoria is one of the problems of rehabilitation and it has long been recognised by the medical profession that such facilities are of great value in the patient's treatment and convalescence. Such training must be designed to ensure that the patient is not allowed to feel he is isolated from normal life or is different from his friends and neighbours. The British Council for Rehabilitation operates a Preparatory Training Bureau which arranges in hospital or at home for (a) practical and theoretical training in technical crafts; (b) study and coaching for entry to the professions; (c) study in authentic courses under University authority. Training has been arranged in respect of such widely different subjects as: accountancy, commercial art, dressmaking, dentistry, embroidery, hospital administration, watch repairing, radio engineering, and teaching.

The Rt. Hon. Ernest Bevin, M.P., when Minister of Labour and National Service in the Coalition Government, promoted the Disabled Persons Corporation Limited, now Remploy Ltd., in accordance with Section 15 of the Disabled Persons (Employment) Act, 1944, and invited the Rt. Hon. the Viscount Portal to be Chairman. The Corporation, formed in accordance with the Companies Act, 1929, is limited by guarantee and is financed by the State. It has no share capital and is non-profit-making.

The function of Remploy Ltd., is to provide employment in special factories or workshops, and, in the case of the home-bound, in the homes, for all classes of registered disabled persons who are so severely handicapped by disablement as to be " unlikely, either at any time, or until after the lapse of a prolonged period, to be able otherwise to obtain employment." In accordance with Section 16 of the Act, preference will be given to disabled ex-Service persons, that is to say, men who have served whole time in the armed Forces of the Crown, or in the Merchant Navy, or in Civil Defence, and women who have served whole time in any of the capacities mentioned in the First Schedule to the Disabled Persons (Employment) Act, 1944. Employment is provided in factories known as " Remploy Factories " and is of a type suitable for severely disabled persons. Training is provided in wood, plastic, leather and light assembly work, etc. Wages are paid during the period of instruction as well as for subsequent employment on productive work. The recognised full trade union rate in each district is paid to disabled persons who are regarded as competent in their work. Travelling expenses are refunded to disabled employees. For those severely disabled, who because of their disability are unable to travel to and from a factory, home work is provided. The products of the factories are sold and bear the name " Remploy ". Subcontracts are undertaken for local industries. The pioneer work at the Papworth Village Settlement and Preston Hall has received well-deserved recognition and the Ministry of Labour and National Service has arranged for financial assistance to be available for the development of these establishments.

Of particular interest to public health nurse are the homework schemes which are a logical outgrowth of Remploy Factories. " Homebound " patients who are unable to make the journey to and from the factory are trained under these schemes to work at home and satisfactory results are being obtained. Perhaps in this field, particularly, the district nurse can make her contribution in that she can suggest and encourage her patients to undertake the training required. Although at first the financial return may not always appear adequate, yet the therapeutic value of occupation, and the fuller interest in life which will grow from it, is recompense enough to justify the thought which is being put into the development of these new fields of social work. Throughout the wide field of social service for disabled men, women and children, which has grown up in this country, the pioneer work done by the voluntary societies is now receiving well-deserved recognition because, although the State is now developing a national "rehabilitation" service, the experimental stages have been quietly progressing through the past century, under their auspices.

It would be wellnigh impossible to mention all those organisations who have blazed the trail in this field, though the Shaftesbury Society by its work for cripples, the British Legion, the National Institute for the Blind, and Lord Roberts Memorial Workshops should be mentioned. Much, however, remains to be done and encouragement is now given generally by the Ministry of Labour and National Service to voluntary bodies who are willing to initiate work along these lines.

2. *Industrial Nursing Service and national economy—a contribution from the insurance world.*

It is possible that the nurse in industry gives little attention to the economic results of her work. She is subconsciously aware that through her prompt attention to accidents, however slight, not only is there a saving of human suffering but also a real economy in manpower at a time when every ounce of energy is essential for the country's recovery. She cannot always give figures to prove her theories. These are, however, not far to seek and the following table compiled from the Annual Reports of the Chief Inspector of Factories shows the trend of reportable accidents. These figures reveal a high average of 40 persons injured for 1,000 employed per annum. This does not include the large number of minor injuries which there is no statutory obligation to report.

In order to assess loss in production it is usual to arrive at an average figure of loss of expectation of working life. This is assumed to be 50 years—that is from age 15 to 65 years. If six weeks is taken as an average disability period for all accidents other than fatal, this is low as it does not take into account permanent and total disablement cases. It is proposed, however, for the convenience of simple illustration to take an even lower figure of 5·2 weeks if for no better reason than that it is one-tenth of a year. In terms of man-years, then, we have the following calculations:

Year	Fatal Accidents	Non-fatal Accidents	Estimated No. Employed
1938	944	179,159	5,590,000
1941	1,646	269,652	6,560,000
1943	1,221	309,924	7,000,000
1946	826	222,933	6,000,000
1948	861	200,225	7,848,000

This means men and women are disabled by industrial accidents to the extent of at least 1,000 per day. If a low figure of say £250 per annum. (i.e. £4 16s. 6d. per week) is taken as an average wage, the annual loss of production can be valued at £25,000,000. This is a simple direct loss and one which, if allowed to continue, might hold up the recovery of the country for many years.

Furthermore, on the basis that £10,000,000 is paid annually in compensation it would be fair to suggest that the hidden costs of accidents, where injury is caused, might be £20,000,000 without taking into account that many items in the hidden costs would be repeated in the 20 to 1 ratio of cases where no injury is caused. The hidden cost cannot be less than £25,000,000 over the whole range of accidents. Thus in full the whole bill annually cannot be less than £50,000,000.

So far little has been said about Insurance Companies and although the nurse has only occasional personal contact with this field, which permeates every avenue of human endeavour, yet her day-to-day duties both directly or indirectly influence their policy. It is, perhaps, surprising that this country, steeped in the insurance tradition both at home and abroad, should have been so conservative and tardy to awake to the great opportunities before them. It is hard to find reasons why they have not adopted a more active and progressive role in the reduction of the risks they undertake and to pass on the public the specialised knowledge they have acquired. In the field of fire insurance there is no doubt that the Fire Offices have made a great contribution to the prevention of fire risks but in the field of human life much remains to be done by other branches of insurance. It has been estimated that 85 per cent of the accidents reportable to the Factory Inspector are due to causes which can be controlled by legislation. But the human element is always present and as an unknown quantity it unconsciously defies all the guarding and safety gadgets which can be devised through the ingenuity of the engineer. This can only be controlled by education of the workers, and in this respect the industrial nurse plays an important part. Through better supervision and safety organisation and by greater care in factory and machine design, industrial accidents can be prevented.

It may be argued that this question is far removed from the nurse in her medical department. But space is being given to it in this history of industrial nursing because the insurance world is at last emerging from its isolated seclusion and is facing reality by practical and experimental methods. The nurse is taking her rightful place in these. The insurance world accepted long ago that the prompt payment of insurance claims on the one hand and the medical supervision of the injured workman on the other were remedial steps only, but were not ready to deal with the hard core of the problem which was the actual prevention of industrial accidents and industrial disease.

First in the field in this country was the Midland Employers'

Mutual Assurance Co. Ltd., with headquarters at Birmingham, which established a special department for the prevention of accidents—a service somewhat similiar to that given by many insurance companies in the United States of America where the prevention of accidents has received, for a long time, the attention it deserves. To quote from a report of this Company's activities the following gives some idea of the scope of the service offered: " Wherever this service is given, in works or factory, one of the department's engineer-surveyors makes a thorough survey of all plant and equipment with special reference to any hazards that may exist. Advice and discussion take place upon points of immediate importance and this is followed by a detailed list of recommendations. In the case of a large works this may run into many hundreds covering such points as the effective guarding of machinery and such items as lighting, hygiene and the highly important subject of protective clothing. Another phase of these activities has been the giving of advice and assistance on the formation and functioning of Works Safety Committees, and in all cases where our policy holders are liable to prosecution for infringement of the Factories Act. . . .

" Unfortunately, injury is not the only physical risk run by the industrial workers. There is the equally pressing problem of industrial diseases. Here again, by timely advice, we have endeavoured to reduce the incidence and we hope eventually to eliminate the hazards that exist. We believe, however, that until each worker, and particularly the newcomer, is given an initial medical examination followed by others at regular intervals, the question of these occupational diseases will continue to be one of the outstanding problems of industry."

In all these new activities the nurse will play her part and from experience it is interesting to pay tribute to the work of this Company whose officers have recognised the function of the industrial nurse in accident prevention in the factory and have actively co-operated with her in this particular field.

Prior to the introduction of the Industrial Injuries Act which followed the former Workmen's Compensation Act this Company maintained surgeries where patients, on claim, were seen by their medical men. The serpent entwining the fasces which is a symbol of healing, through the allusion to the Roman god of Medicine Aesculapius, is a part of the Company's coat of arms and recalls its pioneer work in this direction.

In another direction the recognition of this same obligation by insurance is being expressed by the Crusader Insurance Company Ltd. For many years the Company has encouraged the development of industrial nursing through its Nursing Consultants, who are State-registered nurses with public health and social work experience. A Health Advisory Service now operates not only for its adult and juvenile sickness and accident policy holders but also for factories and other establishments insuring under a group policy. Comprehensive though the National Health Service is, there are gaps and loopholes and the voluntary aspect of the work gains in importance in consequence. This is particularly evident in the fields of rehabilitation and care of the disabled. Among the factory groups insured by this Company, close contact is kept with industrial nurses employed there. Information can be supplied on particular social problems; visits are made by the Nursing Consultants to discuss the development of new activities; encouragement is given to increase co-operation between the industrial nurse and the other members of the public health nursing and social work team; official and other interesting literature is circulated and efforts made to stimulate and develop industrial nursing on broad comprehensive lines.

3. *Continued Education in Industry.*

The first Factories Act of 1844 required that children employed in factories should receive part-time education and early " welfare " efforts were characterised by the introduction of a certain amount of schooling. Not until 1870 was compulsory education introduced. The 1914-18 war drew attention to the urgent need for a new and better world and public opinion was focused on the period between school life and the entrance to industry, this being the vital turning point in child life.

A departmental committee was set up in 1916 by the President of the Board of Education and presided over by the Rt. Hon. J. Herbert Lewis to enquire into "Juvenile education in relation to employment after the War". The Committee started its task with the following statement:

In the great work of reconstruction which lies ahead there are aims to be set before us which will try, no less searching than war itself, the temper and enduring qualities of our race; and in the realisation of each and all of those, education, with its stimulus and its discipline, must be our standby. . . .

Whether we are to be such a nation must now depend largely upon the will of those who have fought for us, and upon the conception which they have come to form of what education can do in the building up and glorifying of national life.

A searching enquiry was made into the conditions of juvenile employment which ranged from well-organised apprenticeship schemes to the blind-alley occupations and other undesirable trades. The report called attention to these conditions as "gravely disturbing". An important forward step was later made by the "Fisher Act" of 1918 which permitted the establishment of Day Continuation Schools and in 1920 such schools were inaugurated at Stratford on Avon, Rugby, Birmingham, Swindon and some few other places.

Industry played its part in the development of further education and one outstanding example of this is the Day Continuation School which has functioned since these days at Nottingham in the firm of Boots the Chemists. This is now known as Boots' College. A very close connection has been maintained between the Nottingham Education Authorities and the Company, and the school doctors appointed to supervise the health of the young people are the medical officers of Boots Pure Drug Company. All minor defects disclosed at the medical examinations are followed up by the school nurses and treatment arranged for their correction. The school nurse holds a clinic twice a day in the school, which is in the factory premises.

All the employees under 18 years of age attend classes one day a week, and health education plays an important part in the school syllabus. The following is an outline of this subject as taught by the school nurses:

1. Talks on personal hygiene and general rules of health are given each term to the new girls—classes slightly varied to suit average age and size of class.
   Posters and blackboard, Agar cultures and microscope used.
2. Home Nursing classes given to the older girls about once a year. This includes two theoretical classes covering:
   Symptoms of an ill patient, observation of an ill patient, nursing at home, keeping patient happy, etc., disposal of faeces, urine, etc., use of bedpan, etc., reporting to the doctor on patient, etc., etc.
   Practical classes on:
   bed-making, sheet changing, lifting, washing, laying of trays, reading of thermometer, etc., treatment of mouths.
3. Classes with senior girls on bacteria, modes of and prevention of infection illustrated by microscope and Agar cultures— how to combat infection in the home, illustrated by treatment of a common cold, cuts and minor accidents at home—on home first-aid box—symptoms of and treatment of shock.
4. Follow-up work on all juveniles is used as an opportunity for individual advice, etc.
5. The social side of the College activities is emphasised by the nurse who joins in such activities as fancy dress dances and school sports.

The Education Act of 1944 is important as a measure seeking to deal with the same problem of juvenile employment as those of its predecessor, the " Fisher Act ". County colleges will one day be established by education authorities and since April 1, 1950, all young persons over compulsory school age and under 18 years of age, unless attending a full-time course of instruction, have continued education. There can be no doubt that industry will again take its place in developing these new educational plans and this question is mentioned in this history because it affects and will continue to affect the work of the industrial nurse. How much she will be able to participate in the class teaching which will be developed is not yet known, but wide opportunities will emerge for close co-operation between the theoretical side as taught in school and the practical side of health education as it will be approached by the industrial nurse in the day-to-day work of the factory.

4. Industrial Nursing Service develops overseas.

The romance of industry in Great Britain is a story which will perhaps one day be written in full, and the rapid rise of many well-known firms within the span of two or three generations of ownership will make fascinating reading. Equally interesting will be the story of the development of health and social services within those industries. It is not possible within the scope of this short history to make more than a passing reference to the wide expansion of international trade since the war years. The economic condition of this country needing an increase in export trade, the heavy burden of taxation and the trend towards a policy of building factories overseas for such reasons as proximity to the raw materials or because of import regulations, has had one immediate effect on industrial nursing. This is the development of health services in other countries of a standard following closely to the pattern worked out at the parent firm.

To illustrate this point, the growth of Lever Bros. and Unilever Ltd. can be described. To simplify nomenclature Unilever is used as a diminutive to identify two sister companies, Lever Bros. and Unilever Ltd., of England and Lever Bros. and Unilever N.V. of Holland. Unilever springs from three principal sources, the Dutch family concerns of Van den Berghs and Jurgens and the English concern of Lever Bros. Each can unfold its own story of the romance of trade. The firms concerned are established in America, Australia, Belgium, Belgian Congo, Holland, India, Pakistan, New Zealand, South Africa, Thailand, Burma, Canada, Ceylon, Denmark, France, Germany, Newfoundland, the Philippines, Switzerland and the West Indies.

With headquarters in London, the Medical Service is administered there. In 1948 Miss E. M. Gosling, S.R.N., Industrial Nursing Certificate, was appointed as the first Principal Nursing Officer. Miss Gosling, who assists the Principal Medical Officer in establishing the nursing policy for the organisation, is an adviser to the management on all matters connected with the employment of nurses. This advisory service is not limited to the United Kingdom but is also given to managements overseas.

Unilever has 73 factories in this country employing approximately 47,000 people. The policy of the Company is to ensure that, where numbers warrant it, State-registered nurses are employed. State-enrolled assistant nurses and female first aid assistants are also employed and work under the supervision of the State-registered nurse.

In all countries of the world where there are well-established factories within the Unilever organisation, medical and nursing services have been established in accordance with local laws and customs.

The story of achievement in the field of industrial medicine by the Anglo-Iranian Oil Company showed steady growth over a period of forty years from 1909. A programme for housing and health was developed at Abadan on the banks of the Shatt-el-Arab. In the tropical heat of south Persia a complete hospital service was established, staffed mainly by European doctors and nurses.

In the field of preventive medicine the accomplishments

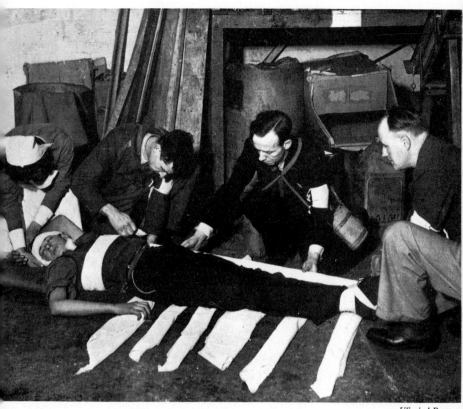

THE INDUSTRIAL NURSE AS A TEACHER

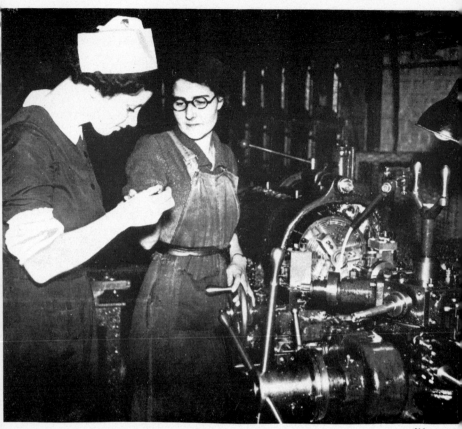

INSPECTION ON THE JOB

of the Company have been outstanding. Diseases such as typhus, malaria, trachoma and smallpox are widespread and constant war must be waged to keep them in check. Extensive "oiling" of stagnant water to prevent the breeding of the malaria-carrying mosquito is a preventive measure which must never cease during the breeding season. These measures were carried out unremittingly by teams of men employed by the Company from early spring to autumn. The use of the modern drug mepacrine for the entire population was introduced and insecticides such as D.D.T. were provided in enormous quantities throughout the whole country. Vaccination against smallpox was also made available to the general population in the area.

Industrial nursing in Persia was truly an experiment in social medicine. The Anglo-Iranian Oil Company's clinics at Abadan were attended by children suffering from trachoma and other debilitating diseases. Persian mothers too, who were helped by the nurses both in hospital and clinics to understand the rudiments of personal hygiene, nutrition and child care, benefited by the wide interpretation put by the Company on their responsibilities. Their programme had not only turned the arid desert into a comparatively healthy place but had brought to Persians an up-to-date industrial health service.

Although the Anglo-Iranian Oil Company has now withdrawn from this scene of operation their work over the years will have left behind a higher standard of industrial health than was found before their arrival.

The Overseas Food Corporation.

The Government venture into food production led to the establishment of the Overseas Food Corporation which is centred in three districts in Tanganyika Territory—at Kongwa, 300 miles from Dar es Salaam in the Central Province, at Urambo in the Western Province and at Mkwaya and Nachinwea in the Southern Province. The part nurses have played in the Ground-nut Scheme in East Africa must take its place in this chapter as it is a post-war development of considerable importance.

The work is naturally based on the hospitals and at the end of 1948 beds to accommodate 576 Africans and 116 Europeans were available. Out-patient departments looked after the needs of large numbers of native employees, many of them suffering from malnutrition, avitaminosis, dysentery, yaws, malaria, trachoma and other tropical diseases. The Health Visitors employed by the scheme find a vast field of work among both native and European women and children. The service is administered by a Principal Matron, Nursing Sister and Nursing Orderlies, the latter having been recruited from all over East Africa and trained by the Corporation's Medical Training School. It is the policy of the Corporation to teach and use English for technical subjects but knowledge of Swahili is necessary for conversation with servants, labourers and children.

Here, then, is a new development of industrial nursing, based upon the widest concept of social medicine which may be destined to have a far more comprehensive appeal overseas than in this country, where specialisation has been developed over the years. It may be the pattern on which occupational health services of the future will be built up in all under-developed territory.

Because of a change in Government policy, all the work developed by the Overseas Food Corporation except the small hospital at Urambo has now been handed over to the Tanganyikan Government.

Among many other British companies which have gone overseas is the English Electric Company with headquarters at Stafford, which controls manufacturing establishments in Australia and Canada. In Brisbane the company has to conform to the conditions of the Queensland Factories and Shops Act. This requires a suitably equipped first aid post, manned by a holder of the St. John Bronze Medallion, to be maintained. The Act also lays down that where a factory employs 300 or more employees, a trained nurse on a full-time basis must be in attendance. The Queensland Ambulance Transport Brigade is available for conveying a patient to the nearest public hospital for treatment. In New South Wales there is a similar Factories and Shops Act which was first enacted as long ago as 1912 and requires that a first-aid ambulance chest must be available in every factory. A further regulation introduced in 1928 specifies the minimum content of the chest for factories of various sizes. This Act does not make a specific regulation that a trained nurse must be available in factories above a certain size. It is, however, the general practice in larger factories to employ a nurse on full-time duties as her function widens considerably as the size of the factory increases.

In Canada the English Electric Company, employing 1,000 employees, and the John Inglis Company employing 1800, both based on St. Catherine's, Ontario, maintain plant hospitals which are fully equipped to deal with any occupational accident. The English Electric Health Centre consists of a waiting room, treatment room, offices for doctor and nurse and rest room with direct access so that ambulances can drive straight to the centre from the street. It is staffed by a full-time nurse and a doctor who calls once a day but is available at any time during plant operations. When an employee is engaged by the firm, he is given a complete medical examination. Results of the examination are entered on a record card, a copy of which is sent to the personnel office and also to the foreman of the department where the new entrant will work. This record states any disabilities the man may have and any jobs or movements which he should not carry out. The Company prides itself on its employment policy of no discrimination against elderly and disabled people. Employees can make full use of the health centre and can consult the doctor at any time, both on occupational and non-occupational illness. Occupational illness or injury will be treated free of charge but advice only can be given in other circumstances. Annual mass radiography is carried out by a mobile unit and any employees who need further X-ray examinations at regular periods are sent to the St. Catherine's Sanatorium, to which the firm makes an annual contribution. The sanatorium is also prepared to X-ray any employees before they are put on the payroll. All English Electric employees are able to make use of the Health Benefit Plan, which is a voluntary form of health insurance. By making a regular weekly payment, which is deducted from the pay packet, they receive insurance cover for all surgical (not medical) bills and also compensation for loss of pay through absenteeism through illness, the payments starting on the eighth day of absence. This is a great benefit to the employees, and is worked through one of the Canadian insurance companies. If an employee is ill, he is expected to produce a certificate of illness signed by a doctor if he is absent for more than three days. However, this rule is not strictly enforced. In the case of minor ailments it is left largely to the factory doctor or the nurse's discretion as to whether the employee should have a certificate or not. Should an employee be absent for more than eight days, for any reason of illness whatsoever, it is obligatory that he reports for a physical check-up with the doctor, to ensure that he is still in a fit condition to continue his work. The John Inglis hospital is staffed similarly to the English Electric Health Centre, with the addition of a St. John Ambulance first aid man who takes over for the night shift.

Industrial nurses in Canada have one great advantage as yet denied the professional in this country. In Ontario a Division of Industrial Hygiene is part of the Department of Health and Nursing Consultants are appointed to this division. Their function is largely educational and advisory and matters referred to them by industrial nurses in the field are dealt with by those who are familiar with the practice of industrial nursing. In Ontario also, a news letter is published and circulated among nurses working in industry in the province. As a means of stimulating professional organisation and raising nursing standards this official publication has an important function in relation to the development of this ever growing branch of nursing in the Dominion.

5. *Spiritual values in Industry.*

Although the immediate stimulus to nursing reform has often been war, it must be accepted that the Christian principles held by those who have been engaged in nourishing and cherishing the victims of war have played an equal part in developing the profession on a firm foundation of Christian ideals. In the nineteenth century religious thought found expression in practical social reforms and was the motive power behind the foundation of many early nursing communities. The band of nurses who went with Florence Nightingale to the Crimea were members of both Protestant and Roman Catholic sisterhoods. Small wonder, therefore, that nursing in Christian countries should have as a common bond the love of mankind and a deep-rooted desire to be of service in distress whether caused by mental, physical or spiritual disharmony.

In industrial nursing these same underlying principles exist in the minds of those engaged there, though perhaps the study of healthy men and women at the bench or at the loom influences the nurse's emotional feelings to a greater or lesser degree according to her personality or background. In the factory she learns to appreciate the dignity of labour but discovers that brotherhood among men and women is not always found among those with whom she works. She believes that man is made in the image of God, working towards a divine purpose and that his soul is immortal, yet she meets him as a cog in an impersonal, inhuman machine, designed for the production of the necessities of life for all and luxuries for the few.

The preamble to the Universal Declaration of Human Rights states: " recognition of the inherent dignity and of the equal and inalienable rights of all members of the human family is the foundation of freedom, justice and peace in the world." In her day-to-day duties the industrial nurse recognises again and again in her own sphere of influence the truth of this profound principle and seeks to interpret its true meaning to those with whom she works. The Lambeth Conference in 1897 emphasised the four principles of Brotherhood, the dignity of labour, justice, and public responsibility for the character of the economic and social order. Subsequent conferences confirmed these principles and in 1918 it was declared that the aim should be " at making the spirit of co-operation for public service with dominant motive in the organisation of industry." In 1930 the Lambeth Conference regretted " we cannot say that society has even yet come to believe that industry exists for man and not man for industry."

Later, in 1942, the Malvern Conference declared the following principles: " The proper purpose of work is the satisfaction of human needs; hence Christian doctrine has insisted that production exists for consumption, but man is personal in all his activities and should find in the work of production a sphere of truly human activity, and the doing of it should be for the producer a part of the ' good life ' and not only his way of earning a livelihood." Indeed, as recently as 1949, the Minister of Education Pamphlet 16, " Citizens Growing Up", published by His Majesty's Stationery Office, re-affirms the same principles. It says:

> The quality of family life depends partly on the beliefs and values honoured by society at large and these in turn are partly created by the standards observed in the homes. From one end to the other, society is charged by the power of ideas and ideals drawn less directly from physical and economic sources than from the spirit of man. All the great religions of the world have attributed to man a spiritual nature and they have linked this, both during the life of the individual and after death with another

and higher order of being. The Christian religion, perhaps more than some others, has concerned itself with social duties on earth. It has exalted the dignity of human personality. It has stressed the brotherhood of man and emphasised the need of good works, as a necessary part of man's duty to God. For Christians, men are brothers because God is their Father and good works are justified not only by their fruits but because they fulfil God's will and contribute to the Kingdom of Heaven. . . .

If homes and schools and society at large are without spiritual ideals, they are houses built on the sand and cannot be relied on to stand against the rising storm.

The labours of Archbishop Temple, who in 1942 invited a group of theologians, business men, trade unionists and economists to consider together the problem of reconciling the structure and practice of the present economic system with the principles of Christian faith, will long be remembered as a great crusade towards a better understanding of a world riven through conflict and misunderstanding. *Man's Work and the Christian Faith*, which is the findings of these conferences written in report form, is a lasting memorial to his faith, wisdom and breadth of vision.

In this country efforts to minister to the spiritual and social needs of factory workers are reported throughout much of early industrial history and in 1877 the Navvy Mission Society was founded by Mrs. Charles Garnett which performed a great work for the Church by means of a trained band of lay missioners who ministered to the navvies and workmen who built the railways, docks, shipyards, reservoirs, sewers and other public works developing throughout the country. The Christian Social Union was later founded in 1889 to challenge the Church to reconsider the teaching of the Gospel in relation to the social, economic and industrial, commercial and political life of society. With this movement were associated the names of Stewart Headlam, Bishop Westcott, Bishop Gore and Canon Scott Holland, who were building on the earlier work of Charles Kingsley and F. Denison Maurice.

In 1919 these two bodies were fused and the Industrial Christian Fellowship was founded under the chairmanship of Dr. H. H. Pereira, Bishop of Croydon. For many years the Fellowship was inspired by the prophetic genius of Rev. G. A. Studdert-Kennedy (" Woodbine Willie "), who did more to commend the Gospel in the market-place, the street corner and public halls of Britain than any other man of his generation.

Much of the work of the Fellowship is evangelical and is carried on by lay missioners who try to reach men and women outside the influence of the Church by means of canteen and open-air meetings in factories, works, mines, docks and throughout rural England. They are also welcomed by working men's clubs and youth fellowships and in other places where men and women gather to discuss the fundamental principles governing the purpose of life and man's relation to it. Dinner-hour meetings are a feature of the work. From time to time an industrial city or a rural area on the invitation of the local Church people is attacked by a crusade of up to a hundred selected people, who carry the offensive into the factories, public houses and clubs in the town. The plan of campaign is not a series of random addresses but a considered statement of the Christian faith and its implications. Generally an encouraging result of this concerted effort brings to the surface a real hunger for the truth and man's yearning for guidance and help. The development of " Industrial Sunday " which is observed in many cathedrals and churches throughout the country is an activity of the Fellowship. On this Sunday, year by year, the Churches are asked to provide a special opportunity to give to men a renewed consciousness that all their activities in agriculture and industry are acts of worship to God. Arranged round the altar, as on harvest festivals, are the fruits of man's labour and these gifts are provided by the neighbouring factories and other industrial activities. Representatives of local government, leaders of industry, and workers' representatives nominated by their colleagues, together with members of the public, join together to give thanks for the industrial harvest in their community. A close link with Industry is kept through the medium of the Fellowship by the appointment, either by the Archbishop of Canterbury or by Industry itself, of chaplains who minister to the spiritual needs of the industrial community. Sometimes leading industries establish a fund for the maintenance of this unusual service.

Into this background of spiritual activity the industrial nurse should find her department merges naturally. In the chaplain or missioner she recognises a friend to whom she can bring those moral and spiritual problems confided to her by her patients. The team is only complete when nurses, doctors and religious advisers can care for their patients together and when they realise how increasingly the interaction of physical, mental and spiritual maladjustment is responsible for much unhappiness in the turmoil of daily life. There are growing up in factory life informal Christian Fellowship groups which are usually small but live cells of Christian witness making their presence felt as a power for good wherever they are found.

Usually monthly meetings are held which are taken by members of the Fellowship and occasionally addresses are given by local clergy and members of the Fellowship or of other Christian organisations. The St. Cross Players also are welcomed by industry to give their plays at special seasons of the year. This unique company of professional artists specialises in presenting religious drama in churches, their stage sometimes being the chancel steps, or the factory hall, specially arranged for the performance. Four tours are arranged each year at Christmas, Lent, Whitsun and Michaelmas, an appropriate play being performed for each season.

A carol service on Christmas Eve, when the whir of the wheels is silenced for a brief period and the Christmas message is recaptured in the old familiar way, is another expression of the same Christian belief. This service is sometimes arranged by the nurse who augments the factory singers by members of the local parish or other church choir. An active part is taken by the Fellowship in any local church effort, and the Christian Commando Campaign and the Mission to London in 1948 found willing helpers within industry for the organisation and follow-up work of those movements to spread the Christian message within their ranks.

In this short history reference has been made before to the wide opportunities for service opening out before the nurse in industry. The horizon is unbounded and although the labourers are few the harvest is ripe and awaiting the reaping.

Conclusion

IT was as a result of a question put by Mr. Ernest Bevin to the Industrial Nurses of the Royal College of Nursing: " What are you doing about India? " that Miss Grace Zachariah came to England to study industrial nursing. The Ministry of Labour and National Service had brought to this country during the war numbers of Indian boys for training in engineering and in their work they had met the industrial nurse and made use of her services. They looked forward to a similiar service on their return to India but expressed the opinion that she would not be found in Indian factories. Mr. Bevin threw out the challenge to the Public Health Section of the Royal College and a scholarship was offered to the Trained Nurses Association of India for an Indian nurse to come to England to study. Miss Zachariah was chosen jointly by the management and men of the Tata Ironworks, Jamshedpur, and besides taking the industrial nursing course at the Royal College of Nursing she travelled widely to see the practical work in a variety of industries. British influence can also be traced to New Zealand, Australia and Finland. In all these countries industrial nurses having qualified at the Royal College of Nursing have risen to positions of responsibility in Government departments dealing with industrial nursing, and in both these Dominions and Finland the work is developing satisfactorily.

The nursing profession was the first women's profession to be organised on an international basis. The International Council of Nurses was established in 1899 and the first postwar review of its progress was in 1947 at the Atlantic City Congress where British industrial nurses made an outstanding contribution to the discussions. The same year a group of industrial nurses went to Sweden for a study tour under the auspices of the Royal College of Nursing and were the guests of the Swedish Nurses' Association. In 1948 the World Health Organisation gave a scholarship for an experienced industrial nurse from Finland to come to England and study at the Royal College of Nursing as preparation for the development of training of industrial nurses in that country.

As this story must come to an end somewhere, 1948 seems an appropriate date for when the first chapter in the development of industrial nursing must close. In this year there were two important landmarks. Up to this time industrial nursing had not been given separate representation on the Nursing Services Committee of the International Council of Nurses. But on the request of the organised industrial nurses within the Royal College of Nursing (one of the professional bodies affiliated to the National Council of Nurses of Great Britain and Northern Ireland) made to the International Council of Nurses the industrial nurse now finds herself represented within her profession at international level.

The other outstanding event was the Ninth International Industrial Health Congress of the Commission Internationale Permanente pour la Médecine du Travail which was held in September in London to which over 900 delegates, at least 100 of whom were nurses, from 43 countries came. The nurses came from Great Britain, Finland, Belgium, Canada, Australia, Sweden and the United States of America. The industrial nurses of Great Britain were invited to assist in the arrangements of the Congress and two Sessions were devoted to their subject, when papers showing the high standard of industrial nursing practice and a wide vision of the educational needs of this growing profession attracted considerable attention. At the Royal College of Nursing an exhibition was staged and demonstrations by industrial nurses of modern treatments and procedures were object lessons enough showing the newer trends in the industrial nursing world.

A last memory of this international gathering is of the crowded lawns at Lancaster House, St. James's, S.W.1, during an evening reception given by His Majesty's Government in the United Kingdom of Great Britain and Northern Ireland, with the Minister of Health, the Rt. Hon. Aneurin Bevan, M.P., and the Minister of Labour and National Service, the Rt. Hon. George Isaacs, M.P., as joint hosts. In a secluded corner of the garden, as the westering sun was sinking in a ball of fire, a small group of industrial nurses forgathered and decided to form themselves into an *ad hoc* committee in order to make a request to the Council of the Commission Internationale Permanente pour la Médecine du Travail for official recognition as an industrial nursing group within the Commission.

The International Industrial Nurses' Committee included the following delegates to the Conference:

Miss Blanche Bishop.	Canada.
Miss I. H. Charley.	Great Britain.
Mlle N. E. Damman.	Belgium.
Mrs. Mary E. Delehanty.	United States of America.
Mrs. Gladys L. Dundore.	United States of America.
Miss C. Mann.	Great Britain.
Mrs. Rhodin.	Sweden.
Miss Ruth Saynajarvi.	Finland.
Miss M. M. West.	Great Britain.

And so comes to an end the opening chapter of the history of Industrial Nursing in Great Britain.

Some Important Dates

1556   Gregorius Agricola published *De Re Metallice* in Basle—Mining in Germany.

Early 17th
Cent.   The Crowley Iron Undertakings in Sussex.

1666   Fire of London.

1689   Thos. Savery—first experiments with steam power.

1692   London (Quaker) Lead Company.

1700   Ramazzini's *Diseases of Tradesmen and Craftsmen* published.

1712   Newcomen's Engine.

1730   Spinning by machinery.

1739   Hospital for the Maintenance and Education of Exposed and Deserted Young Children founded— The Foundling Hospital—Captain Coram.

1756   James Lind's *A Treatise of the Scurvey* published.

1769   Duke of Bridgewater's Canal built.

1764   Hargreaves's " Spinning Jenny ".

1769   Watt patented his steam engine.

1770   Arkwright's Water Frame.

1776   Adam Smith's *Wealth of Nations* published.

1779   Crompton's " Spinning Mule ".

1785   Jonas Hanway's *A Sentimental History of the Chimney Sweepers in London and Westminster* published.

1789   French Revolution.

1796   Dr. Jenner. Vaccination against smallpox.

1791   The first Ragged School founded.

1791   Mary Wolstonecraft's *Vindication of the Rights of Woman* published.

1802	The Health and Morals of Apprentices Act.
1811-12	Luddite Riots.
1818	9 years the minimum age and 12 hours the maximum working day in factories established.
1819	Peterloo Riots.
1825	Stockton and Darlington Railway opened.
1829	George Stephenson's " Rocket " runs on Liverpool and Manchester Railway.
1830-40	Sir Seymour Tremenheere—Reports on Mines.
1830-40	Chartism growing.
1831	Chas. Thackrah's *The Effects of the Principal Arts, Trades and Professions on Health* published.
1831	Truck Act.
1832	First Reform Bill.
1832	Cholera Epidemic. 50,000 died.
1833	Robert Owen formed Grand National Consolidated Trades Union.
1833	Factories Enquiry Commission.
1833	Slavery abolished throughout British Empire.
1833	First Factory Act.
1834	Tolpuddle Martyrs.
1834	Poor Law Act amended.
1837	Queen Victoria ascended the throne.
1837	Registration of Births Act.
1838	Steam transatlantic ferry service established.
1839	Education Act.
1842	Mines Act. Sir Seymour Tramenheere appointed Inspector.
1842	Sir Edwin Chadwick's *Report on an Enquiry into the Sanitary Conditions of the Labouring Population of Great Britain* published.
1843	Governesses' Benevolent Institution founded.
1844	Ragged School Union formed. Lord Shaftesbury first President.
1847	10 Hours Act.

1847   Dr. Duncan, first Medical Officer of Health, appointed, Liverpool.

1848   Public Health Act.

1848   Marx and Engels. *The Communist Manifesto* published.

1849   Bedford College for Women founded.

1851   The Great Exhibition, Hyde Park.

1852   Courtaulds—Welfare activities.

1854   Crimean War—Florence Nightingale.

1855   Post Office Medical Service established. Dr. Waller Lewis, Chief Medical Officer.

1855   W. H. Smith and Son appointed a medical officer.

1855   Civil Service established.

1857   Pasteur's papers on Alcoholic Fermentation.

1858   *Great Eastern* launched.

1859   William Rathbone founded District Nursing in Liverpool.

1859   Henri Dunant founded Red Cross after the battle of Solferino.

1859   Florence Nightingale's *Notes on Nursing* published.

1862   Ladies' Sanitary Reform Society at Manchester and Salford began health visiting and infant welfare service, advised by Florence Nightingale.

1863   Charles Kingsley's *The Water Babies* published.

1864   Act forbade a master sweep employing a child under 10 years old.

1865   American Civil War ended.

1867   Workers prohibited from taking meals where dangerous processess were carried on, *e.g.* lead.

1867   London National Society for Women's Suffrage formed.

1869   John Stuart Mill's essay *The Subjection of Women* published.

1870   Education Act.

1870   British Red Cross founded. Incorporated by Royal Charter, 1908.

1872   Mrs. Jeremiah Colman formed Carrow Works Self Help Medical Club.

1874   J. and J. Colman appointed Kate Southall as a welfare worker.

1874   Women's Trade Union League formed by Emma Paterson.

1875   Artisans and Labourers Dwellings Improvement Act.

1875   Chimney Sweeps Act. Sweeps to have annual licence given by police.

1878   Philippa Flowerday appointed first Industrial Nurse, Carrow Works, Norwich.

1880   Employers' Liability Act.

1887   Queen Victoria Jubilee Institute established.

1887   St. John Ambulance Brigade, founded—1893, women attached.

1888   Union of Match-makers.

1888   Match Girls strike. Bryant and May.

1889   Chas. Booth's *Survey of Conditions in the East End* published.

1889   Prevention of Cruelty to Children Act.

1889   Beatrice and Sidney Webb. *Fabian Essays on Socialism* published.

1890   House of Lords Committee to investigate " sweating"

1892   " Health Missioners " first employed by Buckinghamshire County Council, advised by Florence Nightingale.

1893   Sir Chas. Mather's experiment in the firm of Mather and Platt, hours reduced from 53 to 48.

1895   Marconi discovers radio telegraphy.

1896   Vermont Marble Company, U.S.A., appointed first industrial nurse.

1896   Arthur Whitelegge appointed Chief Inspector, Factory Department, Home Office.

1897   The National Union of Women's Suffrage Societies formed.

1898   Dr. (later Sir) Thomas Legge appointed Chief Medical Officer at the Home Office.

1906   Exhibition of Sweated Industries in London.

1906   Workmen's Compensation Act.

1909   First recorded Welfare Conference in London.

1909   Winston Churchill introduced Trades Board Act.

1912   National Insurance Act. Old Age Pensions.

1914-18 The Great War.

1915   Lloyd George became Minister of Munitions of War.

1916   College of Nursing founded. Incorporated by Royal Charter, 1928.

1917   Health of Munition Workers Committee.

1918-28 Enfranchisement of Women.

1932   Conference of Royal Institute of Public Health, Belfast.

1932   Survey of Industrial Nursing made by Royal College of Nursing.

1934   Training for Industrial Nursing established.

1939-45 The Second World War.

1940   Ernest Bevin became Minister of Labour and National Service.

1940   Women Power Committee set up by Government.

1946-48 National Health and Insurance Legislation.

1947   National Coal Board established.

1948   Ninth International Congress on Industrial Medicine in London.

1948   Appointed Day. National Health Services Act.

1948   Vesting Day. British Electricity Authority.

1949   Report of the Committee of Enquiry into Health Welfare and Safety in Non-Industrial Employment (Gowers Committee).

1950   Report of a Committee of Enquiry on Industrial Health Services published (Dale Report).

Bibliography

A HANDBOOK FOR INDUSTRIAL NURSES. Marion M. West.

A HISTORY OF COURTAULDS. C. H. Ward-Jackson

ALTON LOCKE. Charles Kingsley

ANNUAL REPORT OF THE CHIEF INSPECTOR OF FACTORIES & WORK-SHOPS for Year 1932 (Including a Review of the years 1833-1932)

ANNUAL REPORTS OF THE CHIEF INSPECTOR OF FACTORIES

AN INTRODUCTION TO INDUSTRIAL PSYCHOLOGY. May Smith

ART AND THE INDUSTRIAL REVOLUTION. Francis G. Klingender

BRITISH CANALS—AN ILLUSTRATED HISTORY. Charles Hadfield

CHARLES DICKENS & EARLY VICTORIAN ENGLAND. R. J. Cruickshank

DYNAMIC ADMINISTRATION. Mary Parker Follett

ENGLISH SOCIAL HISTORY. G. M. Trevelyan

EXPLORING THE DANGEROUS TRADES. The Autobiography of Alice Hamilton, M.D.

FAME IS THE SPUR. Howard Spring

FROM THE LEARNING TO EARNING. P. I. Kitchen

FROM ONE GENERATION TO ANOTHER. Hilda Martindale

GREAT DEMOCRATS. Edited by A. Barratt Brown

" HARVEST " THE RECORD OF THE SHAFTESBURY SOCIETY 1844-1944. Hugh Redwood

HARD TIMES. Charles Dickens

INDUSTRIAL HEALTH—AN INTRODUCTION FOR STUDENTS. R. Passmore and Catherine N. Swanston

INDUSTRIAL NURSING. ITS AIMS AND PRACTICE. A. B. Dowson-Weisskopf

INDUSTRIAL RELATIONS HANDBOOK. Ministry of Labour and National Service

IN MEMORIAM—CAROLINE COLMAN. By her daughter, Laura G. Stuart

INHERITANCE. Phyllis Bentley

JANE EYRE. Charlotte Brontë

JEREMIAH JAMES COLMAN—A MEMOIR. By one of his daughters, Helen Caroline Colman

JOURNAL OF THE INSURANCE INSTITUTE OF LONDON. VOL. XXXVI. SESSIONS 1947-1948

KING COTTON. Thomas Armstrong

LORD SHAFTESBURY AND SOCIAL INDUSTRIAL PROGRESS. J. Wesley Bready

LORD SHAFTESBURY. J. L. Hammond and Barbara Hammond

MAY TENNANT—A PORTRAIT. Violet Markham

NEW TIMES, NEW METHODS AND NEW MEN. V. M. Clarke

NURSING IN COMMERCE & INDUSTRY. Bethel J. McGrath

OFFICE MANAGEMENT FOR HEALTH WORKERS. Francis King and Louis L. Feldman

OUR FREEDOM AND ITS RESULTS, by Five Women. Edited by Ray Strachey

OUTLINES OF INDUSTRIAL MEDICAL PRACTICE. Howard E. Collier

ROBERT OWEN. G. D. H. Cole

SYBIL. Benjamin Disraeli

THE CROWTHERS OF BANKDAM. Thomas Armstrong

THE CAUSE. Ray Strachey

THE EARLY FACTORY LEGISLATION. M. W. Thomas

THE HISTORY OF TRADE UNIONISM. Sidney and Beatrice Webb

THE MAKING OF SCIENTIFIC MANAGEMENT. Volume 1. L. Urwick and E. F. L. Brech

THE PILGRIMAGE OF PERSEVERANCE. Ethel M. Wood

TWO CENTURIES OF INDUSTRIAL WELFARE—THE LONDON (QUAKER) LEAD COMPANY 1692-1905. Arthur Raistrick

SMEDLEY'S PRACTICAL HYDROPATHY (1863)

UNCLE TOM'S CABIN. Harriet Beecher Stowe. 1852

WEETMAN PEARSON. A. J. Spender

WOMEN AND WORK. THE NEW DEMOCRACY. Gertrude Williams

WOMEN AT WORK. A BRIEF INTRODUCTION TO TRADE UNIONISM FOR WOMEN. Mary Agnes Hamilton

WOMEN WORKERS AND THE INDUSTRIAL REVOLUTION. Ivy Pinchbeck

YOUNG PEOPLE IN INDUSTRY 1750-1945. Maurice W. Thomas

Index